SOCIAL HYGIENE IN TWENTIETH CENTURY BRITAIN

THE WELLCOME INSTITUTE SERIES IN THE HISTORY OF MEDICINE

Edited by W.F. Bynum and Roy Porter, The Wellcome Institute

Monica Baly	FLORENCE NIGHTINGALE AND THE NURSING LEGACY
Greta Jones	SOCIAL HYGIENE IN TWENTIETH CENTURY BRITAIN
W.F. Bynum and Roy Porter, Editors	MEDICAL FRINGE AND MEDICAL ORTHODOXY 1750-1850

In Preparation

Johanna Geyer-Kordesch	WOMEN AND MEDICINE: A SURVEY AND A HISTORY
David Hamilton	A HISTORY OF SURGERY SINCE EARLY TIMES
Christopher Lawrence	MEDICINE AND MEDICAL SCIENCE IN THE TWENTIETH CENTURY
Christopher Lawrence	MEDICINE IN THE SCOTTISH ENLIGHTENMENT
Andrew Scull	A HISTORY OF PSYCHIATRY
Irvine Loudon	OBSTETRIC CARE AND MATERNAL MORTALITY 1700-1900
Nicholas Rupke, editor	VIVISECTION IN HISTORICAL PERSPECTIVE
Roy Porter and Andrew Wear, editors	PROBLEMS AND METHODS IN THE HISTORY OF MEDICINE
Virginia Smith	NEXT TO GODLINESS: CLEANLINESS, HYGIENE AND PURITY MOVEMENTS IN BRITAIN 1650-1850
W.F. Bynum, editor	LIVING AND DYING IN LONDON 1500-1900

SOCIAL HYGIENE IN TWENTIETH CENTURY BRITAIN

Greta Jones

CROOM HELM
London • Sydney • Wolfeboro, New Hampshire

Croom Helm Ltd, Provident House, Burrell Row,
Beckenham, Kent BR3 1AT

Croom Helm Australia Pty Ltd, Suite 4, 6th Floor,
64-76 Kippax Street, Surry Hills, NSW 2010, Australia

British Library Cataloguing in Publication Data
Jones, Greta
   Social hygiene in twentieth century Britain.
   1. Social medicine — Great Britain
   I. Title
   362.1′042′0941   RA418.3.G7
   ISBN 0-7099-1481-4

Croom Helm, 27 South Main Street, Wolfeboro,
New Hampshire 03894–2069, USA

Library of Congress Cataloging in Publication Data applied for:

Printed and bound in Great Britain
by Billing & Sons Limited, Worcester.

CONTENTS

ABBREVIATIONS

BMJ	British Medical Journal
BMA	British Medical Association
CAMW	Central Association for Mental Welfare
COS	Charity Organisation Society
DLB	Dictionary of Labour Biography
DNB	Dictionary of National Biography
Eug	Eugenic Society Papers
H of C Deb	House of Commons Debates
ILP	Independent Labour Party
MRC	Medical Research Council
NIIP	National Institute of Industrial Psychology
NFYG	Next Five Years Group
PEP	Political and Economic Planning
TUC	Trades Union Congress
BSHC	British Social Hygiene Council
NCCL	National Council for Civil Liberties
BBC	British Broadcasting Corporation
ICI	Imperial Chemical Industries
MOH	Medical Officer of Health
HMSO	Her Majesty's Stationery Office
LSE	London School of Economics
SFS	Society for Freedom in Science

ACKNOWLEDGEMENTS

I would like to thank the trustees of the Mellon Foundation at the University of Pennsylvania whose generosity in awarding me a fellowship 1982-83 allowed me to complete the research for this book. My thanks extend to the Department of History and Sociology of Science for the hospitality and intellectual stimulation they provided during that year.

I owe a debt of gratitude to the librarians and archivists of the following institutions: the British Library, the London School of Economics, University College London, the Wellcome Institute, University of Pennsylvania, University of Ulster, Queen's Medical Library, University of South Carolina at Columbia, New York Public Library.

I benefited greatly from discussion of my work with Joan Austoker, Charles Webster and from the lively controversies which attended the conference on Eugenics hosted by Mark Adams, Henrika Kuklick and the staff and students of the History and Sociology of Science Department at the University of Pennsylvania in May 1983.

I would also like to thank Charles Rosenberg and William Coleman for their advice and help. None the less, as is usual, I would like to emphasise that I have sole responsibility for the point of view expressed in this manuscript.

In addition I would like to thank my husband Paul Bew for his support and my mother and father, especially my mother who died 12 June 1983 and to whom this book is dedicated.

FOREWORD

This is a study of 'social hygiene' — the notion is apparently a relatively unfamiliar one in the British context, though certainly not in the American or German. The topic is what Grotjahn has called 'social medicine' — the whole area of the comprehensive and intrusive attention to all that pertains to human biological (and mental) well-being. This involves a discussion of a range of themes: reproductive biology and child care; health instruction; dietary advice and control; and housing and mental health.

Not all can be dealt with in this manuscript which cannot and does not claim to be a comprehensive history covering all these areas. Instead it concentrates on a limited and admittedly partial area of social policy. It looks at the intersection between the rising tide of eugenic thought in early twentieth century Britain and part of what Grotjahn called 'social medicine' or 'social hygiene'.

The work is not, however, trying to write the 'secret' history of British welfare by suggesting that the key to understanding its development lies in a history of eugenics. Rather it is trying to draw out the extent to which hereditarian and social Darwinist forms of thought affected a wide range of planning and social welfare groups — each of which clearly retained their own specific and distinct objectives. There are at least two important reasons why this should be done. First, some recent literature has tended to underestimate the influence of social Darwinism. Diane Paul has argued, for example, in a 1984 article on *Eugenics and the Left*:

> It should be noted that some historians have begun to doubt the usefulness of the term 'social Darwinism'. Robert Bannister in particular has argued that the term was invented essentially to slander the people it was applied to and in fact accurately describes the views of very few thinkers. . . .[1]

Recent published work has also tended to describe the eugenics movement as rather more politically and ideologically neutral than in fact it was.[2] This study is an attempt to correct these impressions. It intends to show the extent and influence of hereditarian social thought and describe the actual role of eugenics and eugenic argument in social welfare questions.

In doing this, attention is paid to the existing literature in the field. Richard Soloway,[3] Jane Lewis,[4] John Macnicol,[5] and G.R. Searle[6] have very ably covered some aspects of this subject in recent published work: particularly well discussed have been the fields of birth control, family allowances and social policy, and the eugenics movement before 1914. This text aims however, to stress problems to which these authors have given less attention.[7]

The work sets out to describe the 'social hygiene' movement in Britain from about 1900 to 1960, and to show that it was for its activists a significant alternative to more familiar welfare policies until World War II. It reveals that the members of this movement, many of whom are eugenicists, thought of themselves as progressive social reformers, and were advocates of a 'non-partisan' scientific approach to social problems. The text also argues that the social hygienists were concerned about what they perceived to be the decline of the British 'race'. Along the way it shows how the social hygiene movement connected with other movements such as those for rationalisation and planning. An attempt is made to analyse the ideas, institutions and personnel of this movement: to explain its connections to other movements, its appeal and subsequent decline. The objective is to explore a 'political' domain virtually lost in conventional political histories: social medicine is just about the closest contact that one can have with hapless or needy citizens, and there was nothing shy about its practitioners. The running theme of the book is clear — it is a tale of expertise; indeed a tale of the uninvited expert. Skills, not least scientific skills, are central to this work: the aim is to show the meeting of charity, public services and the scientific mind (as it pictured itself), the whole looking at the social problem, as usual the working class, and taking up that always poisonous topic, 'they' are out-breeding 'us', and thus is society placed in peril.

Notes

1. D. Paul, 'Eugenics and the Left', *Journal of History of Ideas*, vol. 45, no. 4 (1984), p. 571; for a different view, see Greta Jones, *Social Darwinism and English Thought* (Harvester, Sussex, 1980).

2. Daniel Kevles, Annals of Eugenics, pts I-IV, *The New Yorker*, 8 October, 15 October, 22 October and 29 October 1984; see also Michael Freeden, 'Eugenics and Progressive Thought. A Study in Ideological Affinity', *Historical Journal*, vol. 22, (September 1979), pp. 645-71.

3. Richard Soloway, *Birth Control and the Population Question in England 1877-1930* (University of North Carolina Press, Chapel Hill, 1982).

4. Jane Lewis, *The Politics of Motherhood* (Croom Helm, London, 1980).

5. John Macnicol, *The Movement for Family Allowances* (Heinemann, London, 1981).

6. G.R. Searle, *Eugenics and Politics in Britain 1900-1914* (Noordhof|International, Leyden, 1976).

7. With the exception of G.R. Searle's important, but brief essay 'Eugenics and Politics in Britain in the 1930s', *Annals of Science*, vol. 36 (1979), pp. 159-69.

1 INTRODUCTION

Social hygiene is concerned with the welfare of society. On the basis of statistics it follows the phenomena of social life, surveys the population in its various states, observes marriage, studies labour and descends into the slough of despond which is poverty . . . It is the task of social hygiene to prevent diseases of society and to maintain the well being of the civil community. In order to achieve this aim, social hygiene must examine critically the manifestations of social life, trace the answers to their source, and there undertake its regulatory and ameliorative work.

(Edward Reich, *System der Hygiene* (Leipzig, Frederich Fleischer Verlag, 1870-71, 2 vols.) vol. 1, p. XVI, quoted in Rosen, 'What is Social Medicine?', *Bulletin of the History of Medicine*, vol. 21, 1947, p. 704.)

This book is about the relationship between social policy, medicine and ideas about a rational social order in Britain in the twentieth century. G.R. Searle in *The Quest for National Efficiency* and Gary Werskey in *The Visible College*[1] have both noted the pervasiveness among some intellectuals and statesmen of the idea of reforming British society through the application of scientific principles. Certainly, the rhetoric of many British social reformers in the twentieth century has been governed by the appeal to reason, science and efficiency as against irrationality, rule of thumb and waste.

This study is about the practical application of these ideas in certain areas of social life, in particular social welfare and health. It is not a philosophical examination but an historical one. The text focuses on the rise and fall of a group of ideas about public and personal health and the social policies derived from them. It examines the individuals and organisations involved in putting them into effect. This group of ideas will be called social hygiene and their origin and development provide the subject matter for the study.

What is social hygiene? It basically emerged from a marriage between the hereditarian ideas of the late nineteenth and early twentieth centuries and the public health and sanitary reform movement of the nineteenth century. The sanitary reform movement had long been governed by the perception of the relationship between social class and disease. The historian of medicine, George Rosen, dates the modern form of this perception to the experience of urbanisation and industrialisation in nine-teenth century Europe. Rosen points to the importance of the statistical movements in European countries which revealed clearly the geographical and class incidence of ill-health.[2] This perception led to investigation and speculation about the social causes of illness. The conclusions drawn and the remedies prescribed from country to country differed depending on the political and social views of the proponents of public health. To illustrate this point Rosen describes how in the 1840s there arose a school of German medical men around Rudolf Virchow who fused their liberal democratic ideas — later to find expression in the revolution of 1848 — with their zeal for medical reform. Virchow and his colleagues saw the endemic diseases of the early nineteenth century as indications of political and social sickness which could be tackled only by thorough democratisation of society. From this democratic revolution would come the provision of medical care for the poor, the rationalisation of medical practice, including a proper state statistical service, and better medical education.

The political circumstances of Britain in the 1840s were different, but the public health movement there shares some similarities. Both Edwin Chadwick and Southwood Smith, its dominant figures, welcomed the growth of urban, industrial capitalism whatever reservations they may have had about some of its effects.[3] Their aim was to rationalise the principles of government, to remove waste, inefficiency and cor-ruption — faults they associated with the 'old order'. The reform they proposed they believed to be perfectly compatible with the free market and the principles of political economy. In fact, they considered they would make the operation of the free market more effective. In other words, public health in both Britain and Germany in the early nineteenth century was strongly intermixed with the values of industrial capitalism. It saw itself as reforming, innovative and sometimes even revolutionary in its impact.

In the nineteenth century under the terms 'public health' and 'sanitary reform' a comprehensive programme of health reform was being advanced. Health reformers included housing, sanitation, nutrition, industrial occupation, infant and child care, domestic and personal cleanliness and mental health in an integrated programme for improving social health, particularly among the poor. In the 1900s the emerging mental sciences and eugenics were added to this programme. The term 'social hygiene' also began to be used, particularly in Germany. In the USA the term 'social hygiene' became eventually a euphemism for sexual regulation and the control of venereal diseases but this was not the case in Britain and elsewhere. By the 1900s social hygiene was written and spoken about as a set of public health reforms which included a strong eugenic component and, increasingly, the mental sciences. Like its predecessors it strongly reflected the social and political climate of the time. Assumptions about health, society, politics and the economy were intermeshed. As the second, third and fourth decades of this century succeeded the first, changes occurred in nomenclature and emphasis. Social medicine became a more popular term than social hygiene and eugenics was given less prominence.

Sir George Newman, Chief Medical Officer at the Ministry of Health 1919-35 noted in his recollections this broadening of the interpretation of health in the period 1900-14. This saw 'an ever-widening interpretation of preventive medicine in relation to the health of the individual and the people', a movement he characterised as towards 'personal and positive hygiene'.[4] Something of this greater role for public health is expressed in the outline of aims published by the newly founded Ministry of Health in 1919. This included the traditional role of prevention of infectious diseases, sanitation and food supply, research and education. But it also included

(1) *A sound foundation of physique* (eugenics, heredity and race, racial poisons including venereal disease).
(2) Maternity and the care and protection of the function of motherhood (Maternity and Child Welfare Service).
(3) Infant welfare and the reduction of infant mortality.[5]

This work, therefore, looks at social hygiene as an emerging set of ideas in one particular historical period in Britain. It claims to do no more. It acknowledges that some of the programme of social hygiene was anticipated by previous public health movements and some remained incorporated under different nomenclatures in succeeding decades. Nevertheless, it looks at the dynamics of, and historical influences producing, a set of ideas about society's health at one particular historical moment, and also at the subsequent decline and, if not fall, at least attenuation of that particular set of ideas.

Because social hygiene involved a whole complex of practices and ideas encompassing individual, family and industrial health, it is a very wide subject indeed. Many aspects of it are not treated here. The issues of birth control, maternity and child welfare and the spread of mental testing have been covered in recent works which have noted the persistence of hereditarian ideas in these areas of social policy. What this work tries to bring out and identify is the exact importance and extent of hereditarian ideas and the reasons for their emergence. Therefore it cannot provide a detailed administrative or social history of all the agencies which could be said to be bearers of the practice of social hygiene in twentieth century Britain. For example a comprehensive history of the mental hygiene movement in Britain and its international ramifications is outside the scope of this study. Nor can the work be a totally inclusive guide to the complex network of organisations that touched on health. Sir George Newman in *The Building of the Nation's Health* lists twenty-eight voluntary organisations alone which sprang up between 1872 and 1935 as well as ever-multiplying state agencies of health.[6] Some of these voluntary agencies are discussed in subsequent chapters and others would deserve a closer examination from the point of view of the thesis in this book. But a comprehensive picture of the work and activities of all these is impossible.[7]

This work deals, in fact, with a relatively limited stratum of middle class reformers many of them situated in peripheral voluntary organisations rather than at the heart of governmental or administrative power. It also fully recognises that the nineteenth century public health movement gave rise to other traditions of reform in the twentieth century which were not social hygienist as defined here — there was, for example, a tradition of philanthropic activity inspired by religious or humanitarian ideals. Protagonists of social hygiene often saw the work of this tradition as unscientific, emotional and even potentially disastrous. At other times they found allies and various campaigns were fought jointly. But ideologically there are clear distinctions. Sir Arthur Newsholme's recollections of his lifelong involvement with public health (he was Chief Medical Officer of Health to the Local Government Board) brings this out clearly. Strongly influenced by Wesleyanism in his youth, Newsholme believed in the transforming power of the cross rather than as he put it, 'mechanical means of improving social conditions',[8] by which he meant birth control.

Newsholme believed in individual moral redemption, which might produce some of the same effects sought by the social hygienist but precluded its methods and assumption. It was drink, Newsholme believed, that lay behind much of the disorganisation and inefficiency of working class life rather than hereditary inferiority. In his book *Fifty Years in Public Health* Newsholme brings this out clearly when he attacks both Karl Pearson and Arthur Balfour for their social Darwinist and eugenic views.[9] Newsholme illustrates the complexity and variety of motives and attitudes behind health reform in the twentieth century.

In addition, though this work deals with the influence of a set of ideas on social policy it recognises that there were pressures shaping it that derived from institutional and administrative developments. The character of medical practice underwent changes in this period and professionalisation occurred in allied groups — full-time salaried medical officers of health, the school health services and educational psychologists. These changes also influenced ideas about health. For example it has been suggested that the rationale behind the experimental Peckham Health Centre in the inter-war years where a policy of comprehensive family care was instituted was, in part, the desire by one of its protagonists to find an enhanced role for the general practitioner in the health service. All these bureaucratic and professional pressures influenced trends in medicine in these years and some of them could modify the conclusions reached by this study.

None the less, given these reservations, the definition of social hygiene in this work allows us to delineate a set of interlocking ideas with considerable influence in this period and with strong roots in twentieth century British society. The text does not attribute universal influence to these ideas about health and social environment but it does argue that a network of individuals and organisations in the first half of twentieth-century Britain subscribed to them. It also argues that their influence on social policy — admittedly quite often frustrated — can be traced. This study examines nutrition, industrial efficiency, social planning, mental hygiene and eugenics. It touches on birth control and family policy in so far as social hygiene encompassed these. It does not aim to give a detailed empirical account of these areas which in some cases has been ably done elsewhere,[10] but to elucidate the concepts underlying the idea of social hygiene and to set out the terms of the debate around it.

When the sanitary reform movement of the nineteenth century tackled the question of ill-health it was, at once, struck by the greater incidence of endemic disease among the poor. This was evident in the great outbreaks of cholera and typhus which affected Europe in the nineteenth century. But investigations had also noted the general relationship between social class and mortality. There were higher incidences of infant and maternal mortality among the poor in nineteenth-century cities. Other studies noted the smaller stature of children from poorer homes as well as their greater debility.

Public hygiene in the nineteenth century and later social hygiene provided a variety of explanations for this. Much, naturally, was attributed to social conditions. But in addition the domestic management and habits of the poor were blamed. Finally and increasingly, towards the end of the nineteenth century, hereditarian explanations were used to account for these social class differences. It was never the case that one explanation drove out the others. They were not mutually exclusive. But it is the case that increasingly heredity was emphasised, and that, out of this change in emphasis, came social hygiene.

One thing remained constant. This was the connection between the eradication of ill-health and economic efficiency. The question of public health was clearly seen by reformers in the nineteenth century as one linked to national prosperity. As F.B. Smith in *The People's Health* points out, Chadwick and his circle saw the prevention of public ill-health as reducing economic dependence and thus increasing productivity. Therefore it would lead, it was argued, to a dimunition of waste and a better work force. As Chadwick put it, it would, 'reduce taxes by preventing disease.'[11] This argument revived strongly in the first decades of the twentieth century. It was encouraged by the sense of national crisis engendered by the European economic and political rivalry leading to the First World War. During the depression of the 1930s, the decline of the birth rate led to similar discussions about the economic importance of a healthy population.

This theme of health care as a form of wise housekeeping was a strong feature of social hygiene. It argued that a little additional expenditure to prevent ill-health would lead, eventually, to a greater saving of money. Governments were not always convinced. But quite often the public were. For example, popular support for the Mental Deficiency Act of 1913 was mobilised by the constant reiteration of the idea that immense savings in the Poor Rate would be achieved by the institutionalisation of the feeble-minded. To this was added, as Colonel Josiah Wedgwood MP protested in his parliamentary speeches against the Mental Deficiency Act, the idea that, with its weakest members removed, the working classes would be made more productive. F.B. Smith argues that if one understands Chadwick's views on the economic importance of health then 'the punitive . . . approach of Chadwick and his fellow political economists to the old and the sick becomes more comprehensible.'[12] None the less whilst this approach might lead to a callous or indifferent attitude to the unproductive, in different circumstances it resulted in attempts to ameliorate the conditions of the healthy poor by better housing, limitation of the hours of work and improved working conditions.

Another enduring legacy of the political economy approach was a conception of health improvement which focused on the individual and domestic behaviour of the poor. Much of the late nineteenth-century investment in hygiene concentrated on moral, individual and domestic reform. This arose from the idea that poverty and ill-health were, where not due clearly to accident or bad luck, self-inflicted. Sturdy individualism, independence and personal provision for old age and sickness were possible for the majority of the working class. The exceptions were those cases where ignorance, weak moral character and bad management intervened. Hygiene was seen as part of the process by which the poor were civilised, disciplined and made into rational economic actors. Thus most programmes of health reform involved personal and domestic hygiene, budgeting and nutrition and the care and rearing of infants, the removal of evil influences and the regulation of the entertainment and leisure of the poor. Such a comprehensive programme implied as one commentator has put it that, 'In this process of civilisation, rationalisation and social disciplining, "health" became a multivalent term of the greatest political potential — from its importance as a guide to living and behaviour, to its importance as the existential basis of wage-dependent sections of the population and finally, its sociopolitical importance.'[13] Such ideas became part of the legacy of social hygiene. They were also, as two recent studies have shown, still remarkably influential in social policy in the inter-war years.[14]

Social hygiene emerged when these assumptions became entwined with hereditarian ideas. By the 1900s in Britain it was common for health reformers to list a series of measures necessary not only for the improvement of individual health but also for social regeneration in general. These included the traditional demands for better sanitation, housing and a lessening of overcrowding in working class homes. It also included measures to combat child mortality by improved means of feeding and rearing children and for the eradication of tuberculosis. Increasingly, emphasis was placed on sexual regulation. This included the prevention of venereal diseases, propaganda about sex hygiene and eugenics. Other social problems, often described as due to hereditary defects, such as alcoholism, vagrancy and feeblemindedness were singled out for urgent treatment. Institutionalisation was increasingly advocated, particularly to control the fertility of the unfit. Claims were made about the possibility of diminishing pauperism through the eradication of mental defect just as it had been popular in preceding generations, and still was, to talk of its eradication through moral reform.

Social hygiene did not separate ill health into sets of discrete problems. Its proponents, whilst they campaigned on various individual aspects of health — tuberculosis, pure milk, venereal diseases, mental deficiency — none the less saw these measures as a portmanteau of social reform. They believed each aspect was related to the other. As George Rosen says of a similar broad approach to health in the USA during the 1900s 'Within such a framework one could attempt to deal with a variety of problems, poverty and dependency, infant mortality, sweatshops, tenements, prostitution and tuberculosis prevention.'[15] Overall, reflecting this broad approach, there was a remarkable amount of peregrination through various areas of health reform by individuals and groups and a high degree of interchangeability between the memberships of different health organisations.

The development of social hygiene must be seen against the growth of state agencies of social welfare in Britain. Until 1908 and the passing of an Act providing for non-contributory old age pensions for the over seventies, the main agency of relief for the poor in Britain was the Poor Law of 1834. This provided for outdoor relief and for indoor relief in the workhouse. It was based on the principle of less eligibility — that is, that relief must not exceed the poorest wage — and, within the workhouse, on a deterrent regime for its inmates. The Poor Law was administered from 1871 by the Local Government Board. The Poor Law also provided for the sick poor through a doctor employed by the Board of Guardians or through one of the infirmaries attached to the workhouses. The Boards of Guardians who ran these were locally elected bodies. The workhouse could include the sick poor, the insane, the feebleminded, orphans, the aged and the able-bodied pauper. However, the majority of able-bodied paupers were relieved outside the workhouse. The local Medical Officer of Health whose appointment, although frequently part-time, was made compulsory for most localities by the 1872 Public Health Act, was responsible for sanitation, infectious disease and adulteration of food, and for regular reports on the health of the community to the Medical Division of the Local Government Board. Leavening this system were innumerable voluntary charities and voluntary hospitals from which the poor and sick might, on application, receive aid.

In private charity the strongest innovatory and administrative force was the Charity Organisation Society which was founded in 1869 in London by the amalgamation of various London charitable organisations but whose influence spread rapidly to other regions.[16] The COS, as it became known, pioneered 'scientific' charity, that is, relief which would be administered in such a way as to lead the applicant to sturdy independence and protect him or her from the degradation of pauperisation. It accomplished this by a careful examination of the home conditions, character and level of self help of its applicants and framed its giving in the light of this information. It pioneered home visiting and its statistical surveys were also a notable feature of its work. The COS remained wedded to the idea of the deserving and undeserving poor. It believed that independence and thrift were well within the competence of the poor — barring unfortunate accidents of fate.

This mixture of government and private agencies was an important feature of social welfare in the late nineteenth and early twentieth centuries. The COS was not the only influential agency of private philanthropy. Most nineteenth-century towns contained a Ladies Sanitary Committee who agitated for public sanitary reform and visited the homes of the poor to encourage or bully the occupants into better standards of hygiene. These committees, formed by ladies of good social position, were one of the pioneers in the development of paid home visitors and they frequently cooperated with the publicly appointed local Medical Officer of Health. He himself was often part-time though this position began to change rapidly after 1900. The Boards of Guardians who administered poor relief to the able bodied and sick poor were elected officials who also served part-time in addition to their full-time occupations. The intermeshing of official and voluntary agencies was an important feature of the British system of health care.

Frank Honigsbaum in his analysis of the development of the Ministry of Health has noted the importance of voluntary organisations. He describes how three hundred voluntary organisations were used by the Local Government Board for the administration of various functions.[17] This tradition continued after the Ministry of Health was formed in 1919 as did the practice of giving grants to voluntary organisations to carry out certain functions subsumed by the Ministry. The Central Association for Mental Welfare and the Social Hygiene Council both benefited from this. These voluntary organisations often pioneered new forms of health care. The maternal and child welfare movement which got under way in the 1890s and 1900s was the result of voluntary efforts. These organisations also acted as an intelligence service. The Charity Organisation Society, for example, was asked by the London County Council in 1890 to conduct a survey of its school population to ascertain the proportion of physically and mentally defective children. The COS was asked to perform other investigative functions, for example to examine the suitability of applicants for free medical care in one London voluntary hospital.[18]

The pioneering, even vanguard role of many of these voluntary organisations in collecting information, hiring paid officials, and formulating policy was increased by what some commentators have seen as the lethargy of government organisations in the period till 1914 and to an extent, thereafter. Davidson and Lowe, in a discussion of innovation in British welfare policy have pointed to the very slow and conservative character of the Local Government Board, which affected the medical department within it and kept it largely subservient to its Poor Law functions. They suggest that the contrast between the Local Government Board and the relatively innovative Board of Trade, which dealt with industrial disputes, was due to the fact that whereas the Local Government Board was staffed by career civil servants appointed through competitive exam, the Board of Trade had a tradition of co-opting experts from the outside. These experts were brought to the attention of the Board of Trade through their writings and participation in voluntary organisations and groups.[19] Consequently, the role of voluntary organisation cannot be underestimated. Whilst by 1919 a central policy organ, the Ministry of Health, existed, retrenchment in the inter-war years still kept government initiative within bounds and innovation was often the result of outside pressure. Davidson and Lowe have pointed to the lack of a proper statistical service in Government in the 1930s. The result was that the intelligence gathering of voluntary organisations and private charities remained important.

The importance of voluntary organisations meant, with a few notable exceptions, a very limited social base from which the health and welfare reformer was drawn. This was important in sustaining some of the attitudes characteristic of social hygiene. It also affected the areas of local government involved in health and welfare where a restricted franchise operated and part-time or unpaid work was the norm. But the situation changed. By 1888 a reform of local government had begun which altered the character of local politics in some working class areas. The Labour politician George Lansbury, for example, had become, by 1892, a member of the Board of Guardians in Poplar, a district in the East End of London and by the 1920s 'Poplarism' had entered the vocabulary to signify a policy of giving relief by need alone and of ignoring the government's calls for retrenchment. Similarly the rise of the Parliamentary Labour Party in the 1920s and 1930s was to influence attitudes. At local level the most vociferous proponents of social hygiene tended to be the institutions unaffected by these developments. But these general political changes eventually began to affect the attitude of voluntary organisations to their role.

According to George Rosen,

It is indeed a striking phenomenon in modern history that the introduction of economic freedom far from doing away with the need for governmental control and regulation eventually led to an enormous increase in the administrative functions of the state . . . even while certain forms of social regulation were being discarded others were replacing them.[20]

The core of the paradox is this, that the more economic restrictions were lifted in the nineteenth century, the more necessary it became to both mitigate the effects of this and, in addition, to discipline, instruct and control the participants in the process. So that for all the COS's talk about sturdy individualism, their work increasingly involved knocking on the doors of the poor, investigating their circumstances, instructing, admonishing and even disciplining them. Social hygiene was truly in this tradition. Whilst social hygiene rejected the idea that the principles of economic individualism were not enough, it became increasingly bound up with regulation and control.

Between the end of the nineteenth century and the First World War the pressures for some forms of regulation, control and reform became stronger. There are various reasons for this, all of them well documented. Bernard Semmel in his book *Imperialism and Social Reform* draws attention to the increasingly collectivist sentiment among many proponents of Empire in this period. Geoffrey Searle has documented the movement for national efficiency among politicians and other writers have traced the influence of these ideas in other social groups.[21] Briefly, much of the impetus for change came from those who, fuelled by the revelations of the poor physique of British Army recruits during the Boer War, believed Britain's Imperial greatness was threatened by the poor physique of her urban working class. These proponents of 'national efficiency', by which they meant Britain's ability to succeed economically and politically against her major competitors, were a force behind demands for certain forms of social reform. In addition, as the literature of this period points out, a section of the Liberal Party were anxious to cement an alliance between the Liberal Party and the working class vote by offering a compehensive series of social reforms.[22] To these forces for change can be added various forms of humanitarian or socialist thought. In this period some socialists were prepared to use the prevalent fears of 'national deterioration' to push for much more substantial changes. This amorphous mass of right wing Imperialists, Liberals, Socialists and 'concerned' people formed a 'public opinion' on the question of social reform in the period 1900-14.

It is interesting to see how this 'public opinion' affected the process of legislative change in this period. Indeed, such an analysis is of particular interest precisely because these changes were by no means all of the same type. Between the 1890s and 1918, especially during the famous Liberal administration of 1906-14, there were a substantial number of legislative reforms. In 1899 an Education (Defective and Epileptic Children) Act provided for special education for the backward child. In 1906 school meals were provided for needy children by the Education (Provision of Meals) Act. In 1907 medical inspection of school children was instituted. The Children's Act of 1908 allowed for the removal of neglected children from their homes. New regulations on tuberculosis were enacted in 1912 providing, under the Insurance Act of 1911, for sanitoria and isolation wards. Regulation on VD was secured in 1916 after the report of a Royal Commission which sat from 1913 to 1916. A Mental Deficiency Act was passed in 1913 providing for the institutionalisation of mental defectives. The war of 1914 interrupted a measure then being discussed in Parliament for the restraint of inebriates. Above all, the 1911 Insurance Act provided several million wage earners, though not their dependants, with unemployment and health insurance. To some extent the Maternity and Child Welfare Act of 1918 helped fill this gap with grants to aid the voluntary 'mother and child' clinics which had grown up before the War. In 1919 a Ministry of Health was formed in recognition that 'health' had emerged as a national concern.[23]

Bentley Gilbert sees this flurry of legislative activity as the result of two processes. The first, covering everything except labour exchanges and national insurance was, he argued, largely above party politics, generally accepted and, though its coming was determined by all kinds of political exigencies, largely inevitable. The labour exchanges and national insurance, however, he sees as the Liberal reaction to the rise of a working class movement particularly the 29 Labour MPs elected in 1906 partly under a Lib-Lab electoral act. Gilbert argues that national insurance, borrowed from the German model, incorporated few of the ideas which had grown up naturally in the British social reform climate and was a departure from consensus determined mainly by the Liberal-Labour political rapprochement.[24]

In fact there was less unanimity even than this. Some of the reforms pioneered by the Liberal government of 1906-14 were much more radical in character than any previous ones, for they departed from the principles traditionally governing poor relief. Non-contributory old age pensions were one straw in the wind, in spite of the fact that political pressure led to the insertion in the Act of a test of character for the recipients of this benefit. The Insurance Act of 1911, whilst it upheld the principle of the individual providing for future events through compulsory saving, offered a non-means-tested benefit. Many social hygienists came from the traditional agencies of charity and poor law work. So that the reforms without a 'test' or which involved state subsidy were felt to encourage the attitude that poor relief was a 'right'.

On the whole the reforms most congenial to social hygiene were those involving medical inspection, control, regulation, instruction and, increasingly, institutionalisation. They saw the purposes of reform in a distinct light. The object was to strengthen the operation of economic individualism not mitigate it. It was also to remove from society, the incompetent and unproductive. Thus whilst sections of public opinion in favour of government intervention came together on many occasions to push for change, it is important to understand their distinct objectives. Honigsbaum draws attention to the coalition of interests which came together to press for the Ministry of Health in 1919.

Haldane's support for the Ministry was expected. He had long been a devotee of medical science and had piloted the NHI (National Health Insurance Bill) through the Lords in 1911 . . . But Willoughby de Broke's support was surprising. He was a reactionary of the old school who had even sponsored a Bill in 1914 calling for the end of NHI and a return to voluntary insurance (with only linked state aid). By 1918 however, he had become alarmed by the fall in the birth rate and this together with a concern for eugenics put him strongly on the Ministry side. Many eugenicists were afraid that Fisher's Bill would raise only the birth rate of the poor and they wanted to help the 'fitter' classes of the nation as well. Under the tutelage of Dr Caleb Saleeby, they had come to see the Ministry as a way of promoting 'radical reconstruction' and attacking the three great 'racial poisons', tuberculosis, VD and alcoholism. De Broke was strongly influenced by Saleeby and his support was extremely important. With him and Astor on the Ministry side, Addison had allies on the right as well as the left wing of the Conservative Party.[25]

In the inter-war years these differences emerged strongly. The principle of insurance became accepted across party boundaries as did the idea of its extension to all in work. But the insurance fund rapidly ran into difficulties because of a continued high level of unemployment and went into crisis in 1931 due to the Depression. Thus the old Poor Law remained, in reality, an important resource for the unemployed when insurance ran out. In 1931 unemployment pay was cut and so were the scales of national assistance (the old outdoor relief). The reaction of the unemployed was hostile and this confirmed the fears of many that a widespread opinion had grown up among the poor that relief should be granted of right and be sufficient to meet all the exigencies of poverty. This was particularly underlined by the resentment at the means test undergone by the unemployed who had run out of insurance.

In the debates on the effect and cure of inter-war unemployment our social hygienists are quite explicit. They accepted retrenchment and when they advocated expenditure, it was for the extension of regulation, inspection, health education and eugenics. They were never really part of the forces building towards the major legislative changes of the 1940s for these were built on different concepts of the causes of poverty, the role of the government, the rights and duties of the poor. In the late 1930s some adjustments were made. But social hygienists were not precursors of the welfare state except in so far as they contributed to its bureaucratic structure. Thus they had heavily invested in a particular view of health and poverty, very strongly rooted in the 1900s, and one of the indications of this was the fascination which eugenics exercised over them.

One of the major intellectual changes characterising the late nineteenth and early twentieth centuries was the growth of social Darwinist thought. There are a great many varieties within this species of thought but two concern us here.[26] First was the preoccupation with external racial and national competition. A recent historian writing of George Wyndham, Chief Secretary for Ireland (1900-5) has commented, 'Like many contemporaries Wyndham viewed a world of competing races in which, using explicitly Darwinesque terminology, only the fittest have survived.'[27] Wyndham was temperamentally and politically opposed to the protagonists of national efficiency although he shared these ideas with many of them. But concepts of this sort were influential among health reformers. Bridget Towers in her article on the National Council for Combatting Venereal Disease has described them as 'endorsing theories which linked the defence of the Empire with the defence of the race.'[28] The second area was the concern with the proliferation of the working class, especially its more improvident members, at the expense of the better stocks. This concern, was not necessarily linked to the former but it sometimes was.[29] In this climate the Eugenics Education Society was founded in 1907. Its history and character, at least until 1914, have been well documented.[30] The social significance and influence of the movement have been less well explored.

Donald MacKenzie sees eugenicists as essentially a middle class professional group, drawn from law, religion and medicine. Very few members, according to his account, came from industry or commerce.

He links the ideology of the eugenics movement to its social character. The emphasis it placed on intellectual achievement, aristocracy of talent, the protection of the standard of living of the middle class and hostility to the working class, he sees as a summation of the social ambition of this stratum. Moreover, MacKenzie considers the Eugenics movement as representing the technocratic and pro-science stream in British life whose natural constituency is precisely the professional classes. Thus MacKenzie sees the Fabians as natural eugenicists.

Eugenics, however, had much wider bases. Like other social hygiene groups it drew its membership from existing voluntary charitable, sanitation and welfare societies. Many of these originated in the 19th century industrial middle classes but by 1900 the social composition of these reflected, as we shall see, a very broad reach of middle, upper middle, landed and even aristocratic society. In addition, eugenics' involvement with capitalism was by no means negligible. The tendency has been to deduce the social character of the Eugenics Society from the London-based Eugenics Education Society. London was, until the inter-war years, largely a commercial and political centre with little large scale manufacturing industry and this is reflected in the composition of many of its organisations concerned with social policy and welfare. For example a recent work on the Manchester District Provident Society (the equivalent to the COS) shows how it reflected much more strongly the industrial character of the region.[31] In contrast the COS in London represented what Gareth Stedman Jones has called 'the urban gentry' drawn from the professional classes, religion, law, medicine and public service.[32]

A similar dichotomy can be seen between the Eugenics Education Society of London and its provincial counterparts. Whilst these often drew upon the 'urban gentry' they also contained networks of prominent industrial and commercial families. In Birmingham, of the 25 members of the Council of the Chamber of Commerce listed by R. Hay for 1906, six had connections with the Birmingham Heredity Society (allied to the Eugenics Education Society) either through relatives or in their own right.[33] In the Birmingham society, apart from these, among its 234 members were the Cadburys, a prominent manufacturing family, Liberal in politics, and the Chamberlains, directors of the Birmingham Small Arms Company, one of the prominent engineering firms in the city, whose politics were Conservative. The society also included directors of the Lyttleton Collieries, R. Cruickshank Limited, Wright Bindley and Gell, Mitchell and Butler Limited and a representative of W. Tangye, the engineering family who owned the Cornwall Works in Birmingham. Similar configurations can be picked out for the Liverpool and

Manchester areas.[34] It was a common mixture in these societies to find citizens prominent in business, the local medical officer of health — for example, Dr John Robertson in Birmingham and Dr James Niven in Manchester — doctors such as Nathan Raw in the Liverpool society and members of local charities and welfare organisations from which the large representation of women were drawn. The eugenics movement was not an exclusive stratum or group. It was a social mix bound together by a set of ideologies about social health.

There are other factors which should revise the idea that eugenics was exclusively a professional middle class creation. At the top levels of British society a great deal of integration and cohesion existed. Alan Kidd says of the original industrial families which dominated the Manchester District Provident Society in the mid nineteenth century that by 1900,

> These men were the heirs of commercial capital which they themselves had not created. Each held a large estate . . . Together they personify the very English process whereby the second generation of any parvenu bourgeois family could be assimilated into the 'upper class' by the vehicle of a public school education . . .[35]

This process is also exemplified by T.H. Marshall, 1893-1981, historian of the British professional classes, doyen of British social policy theory and, after 1945, member of the Eugenics Society. According to A.H. Halsey,

> He was a textbook offspring of the characteristic blending of the bourgeoisie and the gentry in nineteenth century England, with its roots and sentiments in the country, its official place in London, its investments in industry and its occupation in the major professions and higher officialdom. His great grandfather had made an industrial fortune in the north a hundred years before. His family had settled in the Lake District and retained this connection to arcadian affluence from its later London home. His father was a successful architect.[36]

Leonard Darwin the first president of the Eugenics Society typifies this process. The Darwin fortune was, in part, the product of the Wedgwood pottery firm. The Wedgwoods and Darwins intermarried, settled their families on country estates and pursued professional and official occupations. Leonard Darwin himself was an army engineer. None the less this did not preclude a continuing interest in business. In

1908 Darwin was a director of the India Rubber Company, the Gutta Percha and Telegraph Works, Palmer Tyre Limited and the Spanish National Submarine Telegraph Company, in addition to any other income he derived from investment.[37] In 1911 the Eugenics Council contained Sir John Cockburn a politician, director of the Scottish Australian Bank, General Investors and Trustees and the Mount Lyell Mining and Railway Company (London Branch); Sir Harry Cunningham, a judge, director of the American Investment Trust Company, the Chartered Bank of India, Australia and China, and the South Behar Railway Company; and Sir James Crichton-Browne, director of Bovril Limited and the Scottish Widows Insurance Company.[38]

The Eugenics Society was, as we shall see, much more concerned with questions of economic efficiency, productivity and the development of capitalism than the view of it as largely a professional middle class institution might suggest. It certainly benefited from apprehension about low fertility in the middle class and attacks on the middle class standard of living. But there were many groups formed at this time for the defence of the middle class which could be more politically effective in these areas. They included the Middle Class Defence Organisation (1906) and the Income Tax Reduction Society (1907) in addition to many much broader political movements which were anti-socialist and patriotic. The Middle Class Union founded in 1919 became in the 1920s the Grand National Citizens Union. Its anti-red and anti-strike philosophy was orchestrated by Lady Askwith, a very important figure in eugenics in the 1920s.[39] The Union was strongly pro-eugenic and pro-sterilisation. But ultimately eugenics was a means, like the other aspects of social hygiene, of managing the health, moral and social condition of the poor. This, rather than the narrower expectations of a social or professional stratum *vis-à-vis* society as a whole, determined its course.

Notes

1. G. Searle, *The Quest for National Efficiency* (Basil Blackwell, Oxford, 1971) p. 257; G. Werskey, *The Visible College* (Allen Lane, London, 1978).

2. G. Rosen, 'What is social medicine?', *Bulletin of the History of Medicine*, vol. 21 (1947) pp. 674-733. See also William Coleman, *Death is a Social Disease* (University of Wisconsin Press, Wisconsin, 1982), for a discussion of the role of public health reformers in nineteenth-century France and their relation to classical political economy.

3. S.E. Finer, *The Life and Times of Sir Edwin Chadwick* (Methuen and Co., London, 1952); C.F. Brockington, *A Short History of Public Health*, 2nd edn (J. & A. Churchill, London, 1966).

4. G. Newman, *The Building of Nation's Health* (Macmillan, London, 1939), p. 139.

5. Ibid., pp. 434-5.

6. Ibid., p. 446. Among those mentioned by Newman and discussed subsequently are the British Social Hygiene Council (1914), People's League of Health (1917), New Health Society, (1926) National Council for Mental Hygiene (1935).

7. The strong eugenic element in the discussion of TB would make the history of the National Association for the Prevention of Tuberculosis (1899) an interesting study. As late as 1935 the *Manchester Guardian* reported Leonard Hill at the New Health Society's Summer School on Sterilisation as arguing that 'there was one particular disease to which attention should be drawn — namely tuberculosis — which had a strong hereditary background. Consumptives in their own interests but particularly in the interests of the nation, should be sterilised.' *Manchester Guardian*, 3 September 1935.

8. Newsholme, *Fifty Years in Public Health* (Allen and Unwin, London, 1935), pp. 26-7.

9. Ibid., p. 407. Newsholme refers to Balfour's address to the British Association, 5 September 1904.

10. Angus McLaren, *Birth Control in Nineteenth Century England* (Croom Helm, London, 1977). R.A. Soloway, *Birth Control and the Population Question in England, 1877-1930* (University of North Carolina Press, Chapel Hill, 1982). For birth control see Angus McLaren and Soloway; also J.A. and Olive Banks, *Feminism and Family Planning in Victorian England* (Liverpool University Press, Liverpool, 1964). For Family Policy see McLaren and Soloway; also Jane Lewis, *The Politics of Motherhood* (Croom Helm, London, 1980); John Macnicol, *The Movement for Family Allowances, 1918-45* (Heinemann, London, 1981).

11. F.B. Smith, *The People's Health, 1830-1910* (Croom Helm, London, 1979) pp. 420-1.

12. Ibid., p. 421.

13. A. Labisch, 'Doctors, Workers and the Scientific Cosmology of the Industrial World', *Journal of Contemporary History*, vol. 20 (1985), p. 600.

14. See Lewis, *The Politics of Motherhood* and Macnicol, *The Movement for Family Allowances*.

15. George Rosen, *Madness in Society* (Routledge and Kegan Paul, London, 1968) p. 271.

16. C.L. Mowat, *The Charity Organisation Society, 1869-1913* (Methuen, London, 1961).

17. Frank Honigsbaum, *The Struggle for the Ministry of Health*, (Occasional Papers on Social Administration, No. 37, London, 1970), p. 14.

18. F.B. Smith, *The People's Health*, p. 278.

19. R. Davidson and R. Lowe, 'Bureaucracy and Innovation in British Welfare Policy, 1870-1945' in W.J. Mommsen (ed.), *The Emergence of the Welfare State in Britain and Germany, 1850-1950* (Croom Helm, London, 1981), pp. 107-30.

20. G. Rosen, *A History of Public Health* (MD Monographs in Medical History, New York, 1958) p. 225.

21. Bernard Semmel, *Imperialism and Social Reform* (George Allen and Unwin, London, 1960).

22. Among the extensive literature on this topic is Peter Clarke, *Lancashire and the New Liberalism* (Cambridge University Press, Cambridge, 1971); *Idem, Liberals and Social Democrats* (Cambridge University Press, Cambridge, 1978); Michael Freeden, *The New Liberalism. An Ideology of Social Reform* (Oxford University Press, Oxford, 1978); Stefan Collini, *Liberalism and Sociology, L.T. Hobhouse and Political Argument in England, 1880-1914* (Cambridge University Press, Cambridge, 1979); and P. Weiler, *The New Liberalism. Liberal Social Theory in Great Britain, 1889-1914* (Garland, New York, 1982).

23. The history of British social policy is covered in the following works: Derek Fraser, *The Evolution of the British Welfare State* (Macmillan, London, 1973); B.B. Gilbert, *The Origins of National Insurance in Britain* (Michael Joseph, London, 1966); J.R. Hay, *Origins of the Liberal Welfare Reforms* (Macmillan, London, 1975); M.E. Rose, *The Relief*

of Poverty, 1834-1914 (Macmillan, London, 1972); Pat Thane, *The Foundation of the Welfare State* (Longmans, London, 1982).

24. Gilbert, *Origins of National Insurance*, p. 448.

25. Honigsbaum, *The Struggle for the Ministry of Health*, p. 45. Lord Haldane was a prominent Liberal politician. He was an Imperialist and disciple of national efficiency (see Searle, *Quest for National Efficiency*). He was also the uncle of J.B.S. Haldane who figures later in this work. Willoughby de Broke was a member of the Birmingham Heredity Society in 1913. This was affiliated to the Eugenics Society.

26. See G. Jones, *Social Darwinism and English Thought* (Harvester, Brighton, 1980). See also Freeden, *The New Liberalism* and Collini, *Liberalism and Sociology* for the influence of Darwinism on the thought of progressive Liberalism.

27. Andrew Gailey, *The Unionist Government's Policy Towards Ireland, 1895-1905*, unpublished PhD thesis, Cambridge, 1982, p. 154.

28. Bridget A. Towers, 'Health Education Policy 1916-26, Venereal Disease and the Prophylaxis Dilemma', *Medical History*, vol. 24, (1980), p. 72.

29. This fear fed into the birth control movement; see Soloway, *Birth Control and the Population Question*.

30. See Lyndsay A. Farrall, *The Origins and Growth of the English Eugenics Movement, 1865-1925*, unpublished PhD thesis, Indiana University, 1970; G.R. Searle, *Eugenics and Politics in Britain, 1900-14* (Noordhof International, Leyden, 1976); Donald MacKenzie, *Statistics in Britain, 1865-1930* (Edinburgh University Press, Edinburgh, 1981). For the inter-war period see G.R. Searle, 'Eugenics and Politics in Britain in the 1930s', *Annals of Science*, vol. 36, (1979) pp. 159-69; Macnicol, *The Movement for Family Allowances*, M. Freeden, 'Eugenics and Progressive Thought. A study in ideological affinity', *Historical Journal*, vol. 22 (1979) pp. 645-71; *idem*, 'Eugenics and Ideology', *Historical Journal*, vol. 26 (1983), pp. 959-62; Greta Jones, 'Eugenics and Social Policy Between the Wars, *Historical Journal*, vol. 25 (1982), pp. 717-28.

31. Alan Kidd, 'Charity Organisation and the Unemployed in Manchester, 1870-1914', *Social History*, vol. 9 (1984), pp. 45-66.

32. See Gareth Stedman Jones, *Outcast London* (Oxford University Press, Oxford, 1971).

33. See Roy Hay, 'The British Business Community Social Insurance and the German example' in Mommsen (ed.) *The Emergence of the Welfare State in Britain and Germany 1850-1950*.

34. In Manchester, for example, Sir Charles Behrens and Harold Behrens of the family of Jacob Behrens and Sons, Shipping Merchants, were members of the Eugenics Society. In Liverpool, for which the membership list is much more complete, the following were members. G.H. Cox, chairman of the Mersey Power Co. Ltd and Northeastern Salt and Westall; Thomas Goffey, director of Binneys Ltd and Great Wyreley Colliery Company Ltd; the Reverend James Hamilton of Shaw, Hamilton and Company, Merchants, and Anglo-American Oil; W.S. Porter, director of African Merchants Ltd; Edwin Robinson, director of John Prestman and Co. Ltd; W. Oulton, director of Bold Hall Estates, Francis Morton and Co., and Penrhos Colliery Ltd; A. Villar, director of Canadian Mining. The Liverpool Society also included Mrs Edith MacIver, of the family of MacIver Steamship Co.; Mrs Frisch of Eugene S. Frisch, chairman of Pranges Estancis Co. Ltd, River Plate Land and Farming Company; Mrs Thos Guthrie of Guthrie, Balfour and Williamson and Co. Merchants; Mrs Lund of W. Lund and Sons, Shipowners. This information has been arrived at by comparing names and addresses (addresses especially in the case of women) of Eugenics Society membership lists in 1913 with the names and addresses in the Directory of Directors for that year.

35. Kidd, 'Charity Organisation and the Unemployed', p. 54.

36. A.H. Halsey, 'T.H. Marshall, Past and Present, 1893-1981', *Sociology*, vol. 18, (1984), p. 1.

37. See *Directory of Directors*, 1908-13. Also G.C. Allen, *The Industrial Development of Birmingham and the Black Country* (Allen and Unwin, London, 1929) pp. 181 and 303.

See also Eugenics Society membership lists in the annual reports 1908 and 1913. In a random sample of members of the Eugenics Society of 1937, of 164 members resident in the United Kingdom, 17 are listed in the Directory of Directors of that year. When it is taken into account that 56 of the sample were women — therefore unlikely to be directors of companies — the number is not inconsiderable. This is particularly so when the 17 are compared with the 28 of the sample with medical qualifications. By this criterion the medical profession was not overwhelmingly dominant in the Eugenics Society.

   38. Ibid.

   39. Lady Askwith was the wife of a prominent civil servant and expert on industrial relations, Sir George Askwith. Both were strongly anti-socialist. Lady Askwith served on various Eugenics Society committees, including press and propaganda. Her contacts in the press were used by the Eugenics Society during the 1934 sterilisation debate to try to get favourable publicity placed there.

THE TASK OF SOCIAL HYGIENE

> This is the century of Social Hygiene. The time is at hand when we
> shall direct attention to the causes of social ills as in the last century,
> medical men concentrated effort on the prevention of endemic disease.
> (Elizabeth Sloan Chesser, *Women, Marriage and Motherhood*
> (Funk and Wagnalls, New York and London, 1913), p. 183.)

In the first two decades of the twentieth century, concern about the health
of the British population was growing. To some extent this concern was
a continuation of the fears expressed about the nation's health in the nineteenth century. The contagion arising from the slums, overcrowding and
insanitary conditions still absorbed a good deal of attention.[1] But there
are differences. Since the Boer War (1899-1901) revealed the poor
physical condition of the average recruit to the army, there was an
increasing emphasis on individual physical fitness. The growing imperial
rivalry between the European nations increased the fear that British
resources of fit and healthy manpower were on the decline.[2] Moreover,
industry also paid a heavy price for the diseased and debilitated among
the working class. To some it seemed that social progress itself was at
stake.

In 1926 the zoologist, Professor J.A. Thomson, wrote a series of
articles for the *Quarterly Review* describing the relationship between
biology and social life.[3] There were three areas where they touched and
Thomson described these as folk, work and place. Folk covered life itself,
sexual reproduction and the physical and mental quality of the population. Work involved occupational health and industrial efficiency. The
third area — place — concerned the improvement and beautification of
the environment. A few years later, in 1934, Julian Huxley described
biological and social engineering in much the same terms. He believed
that the broad political ideals on which society was founded needed to
be supplemented by science, in particular the sciences of heredity and
psychology. This meant that, in the future, everyone would be subjected
to 'measurement of physique, temperament, intelligence, constitutional
proneness to disease, vocational aptitudes, special gifts.'[4]

In 1912 Havelock Ellis called this movement social hygiene. He used
a phrase which subsequently was adopted by groups combating VD and
prostitution. But in 1912 social hygiene encompassed not only that but
much more substantial changes. According to Havelock Ellis,

it ceases to be simply a reforming of forms and approaches in a comprehensive manner not only the conditions of life but life itself. In the second place, its method is no longer haphazard but organised and systematic, being based on a growing knowledge of those biological sciences which were scarcely in their infancy when the era of social reform began. This social hygiene is at once more radical and more scientific than the old conception of social reform. It is the inevitable method by which at a certain stage civilisation is compelled to continue its own course and to preserve, perhaps to elevate the race.[5]

What did these writers mean? First of all, they saw social hygiene as a concerted attack on a number of recognisable social evils, not simply on discrete problems as they arose. Their writings on these subjects are a comprehensive drawing-in of many, not single aspects of life. Second, they believed that social hygiene meant a more active involvement of the state in social welfare. Third, they thought that, informed as they were by the laws of biology, social hygienists were above the political and social battle. They were like science itself, neutral, uncontroversial and progressive. Fourth, they believed, with Ellis, that whilst this movement was in some respects part of the tradition of nineteenth century social reform, it was radically different in other ways. It was scientific as well as humanitarian whereas previous reform movements had been largely humanitarian. It was also more fundamental, for it brought the regulation of human nature and heredity within the grasp of the reformer. For the first time, psychology and the control of human reproduction were to be allied to the more traditional methods of environmental reform. In an article published in 1911, Elizabeth Sloan Chesser talked of social hygiene in these terms. In her list of necessary reforms, she included better housing and sanitation, purer milk supplies, instruction of the working class mother in the principles of nutrition and the elimination of syphilis, alcoholism, vagrancy, feeble-mindedness. She also advocated certificates of fitness for marriage and the instruction of school-children in the laws of sex.[6]

This book is about the movement for social hygiene examined through the activities of a number of organisations founded in this era. The first of these was the Eugenics Education Society (later the Eugenics Society) set up in 1907. The first Eugenics Education Society was in London but others were formed in provincial parts of Britain and, by 1914, there were Eugenics Education Societies, or their equivalents, in Birmingham, Manchester, Brighton, Liverpool, Cambridge, Edinburgh, Glasgow,

Belfast and Hazlemere. The aim of the Society was to improve the quality of the race.[7] This was to be accomplished by negative eugenics, the prevention of reproduction among 'low quality' human stock, and positive eugenics, the encouragement of reproduction among 'good' stock. Which human stock was good and which bad was a matter of controversy from the very beginning. So too was the idea of science intruding into such delicate areas as the family, and the Eugenics Society was warned of this by the former Conservative Prime Minister Arthur Balfour, otherwise sympathetic to their cause, when he addressed their first conference in 1912.[8] None the less the Eugenics Society became rapidly embedded in an area of British life and remained influential in social policy until the Second World War. The reasons are clear if we see the Society less as an innovation in itself but as a natural consequence of the movement towards social hygiene.

The Eugenics Education Society rapidly moved into several areas of social hygiene. It agitated for the reform of the inebriacy laws, and became deeply involved, in conjuction with the Charity Organisation Society, in the agitation for an Act of Parliament to institutionalise mental defectives. A member of the Society, Mrs Neville Rolfe, founded with the help of the Eugenics Education Society, the Society for Combatting Venereal Disease which in 1925 changed its name to the British Social Hygiene Council. In addition, members of the Eugenics Education Society were strongly represented in other social hygiene organisations.[9]

This is certainly the case with the Central Association for Mental Welfare. This was the successor to the National Association for Promoting the Welfare of the Feebleminded. It was constituted in 1913 as the result of the provisions of the 1913 Mental Deficiency Act. This Act allowed for local voluntary committees to undertake the task of ascertaining the mentally deficient in need of institutionalisation in an area and referring them to the proper authorities for certification. These local mental deficiency committees, which formed the backbone of the CAMW, also provided guardianship for mental defectives who were allowed outside the institution on licence, that is, under supervision. The CAMW although founded in 1913 did not really come into existence until the end of the First World War. Between 1918 and 1939, when it merged its identity with other mental health groups, it was the main organisation concerned with mental deficiency. It expanded its activities during these years into conferences and courses on mental deficiency for medical men and it trained the first social workers in mental health. It also published from 1920 a magazine *Studies in Mental Inefficiency* which changed its name to *Mental Welfare* later in the decade.[10]

Two other bodies concerned with psychology and behaviour came into being in the early 1920s. In 1919 the National Institute of Industrial Psychology was founded with, from 1922, the experimental psychologist C.S. Myers as its first director. This organisation was supported by private grant and donation and did work for industry and government on vocational selection and productivity.[11] The second organisation was the National Council for Mental Hygiene founded in 1922 with Sir Maurice Craig as its president.[12] This was largely composed of medically qualified persons involved in psychiatric or psychological work. The objective which distinguished it from other groups in this field was its interest in 'normal' psychological development and especially in child psychology. But its early interests were also in mental deficiency policy and industrial psychology and it therefore overlapped to some extent with the CAMW and the NIIP.

Two other health reform organisations came into existence in this period. In 1917 the People's League of Health was founded by Olga Nethersole. This remarkable lady had been an actress before turning her attention to the nation's health. According to her own account, whilst compiling a National Register in Southwark, during the First World War, Nethersole had been astonished at the insanitary and unhygienic conditions which prevailed in working class homes.

> I knew that slums breed disease, moral and physical. I was convinced that what Government and human society does not spend on adequate housing and education and protection of workers, male and female, it pays in hundredfold amounts in Hospitals, Prisons, Workhouses, Asylums, Homes for Cripples, Epileptics and the feebleminded. I knew that hundreds of thousands of pounds were contributed annually in this way for the support of defectives, and in comparison how few pounds for the dissemination of the saving knowledge which might prevent it. I had for many years realised that laziness, drunkenness and crime were symptoms of disease and that the trained mind and practised eye alone knew the real meaning of the anaemic, sallow, underweighted, narrow chested, stooping shouldered human with decayed, few or no teeth, faulty eyesight and the true cause of slackness, laziness, minimum power of resistance to disease, moral and physical, and tendency to alcoholic excess.[13]

The People's League exemplified perfectly the broadness of the mandate of social hygiene. It offered general social regeneration through health policy and, though it gradually became more specific in its objectives, it ranged over a wide area of interests. Olga cited eugenics, psychological instruction of youth, control of prostitution, institutionalisation of mental deficients and control of alien immigration along with the more traditional aims of better housing and sanitation as the means to social and Imperial strength. The People's League also believed in the importance of nutrition as did the New Health Society 1926-1937.

This latter Society owed its existence, like the People's League, to a charismatic figure. It was founded by an eminent surgeon Sir William Arbuthnot Lane who had reached the conclusion in his work that much of modern disease was due to defective diet and in particular to 'intestinal stasis'. The foundation of the New Health Society caused a breach between Arbuthnot Lane and the BMA. The latter thought that the New Health Society was too much concerned with the publicising of Sir William's own particular and idiosyncratic medical opinions. None the less the New Health Society attracted considerable support. Sir Lynden Macassey, the lawyer and public servant (famous or infamous for his clash with the Clydeside shop stewards' committee during the First World War) conducted its legal work. Lord and Lady Oxford, the Asquiths, became patrons.

The objects of the New Health Society were to teach the people the simple laws of health, to get fruit and vegetables on the dinner table at reasonable cost, 'to re-settle the people on the land and therefore relieve the misery and hardship due to the overcrowding of big towns'.[14] To this end, a magazine *New Health* was founded and, like the People's League, the New Health Society organised public lectures, tours and summer schools. It was also very much in favour of eugenics. Heredity as well as diet was considered to influence the nation's health and both were considered to have been adversely affected by urban growth. Thus resettlement on the land was intended to do two things, allow a more natural diet and, second, produce the conditions in which hardiness, energy and independence would be selected. This would rid society of the 'discontents and unemployables who clog the wheels of progress, create disharmony and foster revolution'.[15]

The early years of the twentieth century saw a flurry of legislative activity directed at social and medical problems. A number of Royal Commissions and Departmental Committees heralded this legislation. In 1904 the Inter-departmental Committee on Physical Degeneration reported on the causes of the poor health of the nation. This was followed by a Royal Commission on the Care and Control of the Feebleminded (1908), a Departmental Committee on Inebriacy (1908) and many others. Each of these was, of course, aimed at a specific problem but increasingly some general solutions emerged which were considered relevant to a wide range of problems.

In particular institutionalisation was canvassed as a solution to problems ranging from alcoholism to unemployment. Moreover, compulsory not voluntary institutionalisation was advocated.[16] The objective of this was not necessarily rehabilitation or treatment though in some cases it was. For example, the Labour colonies advocated for the able-bodied unemployed, were intended to inculcate labour discipline and eventually return the unemployed to productive work in the outside world. Institutionalisation was also seen as preventing the spread of corrupting influences in society at large. But the doctrine of heredity came to play an important part in the movement for confinement. If social problems were the consequence of hereditary defect, then segregation in institutions was seen as a means of preventing the propagation of the unfit. These eugenic concerns clearly arose in the successful agitation for the Mental Deficiency Act of 1913 and since eugenics, the feebleminded and institutionalisation play such a significant role in social hygiene, it is worth disentangling the issues in that agitation.

The first steps were taken as a result of the Report of the Royal Commission on the Care and Control of the Feebleminded. In 1908 the *BMJ* summarised its findings.[17] The Report advocated a new central commission to look after the following categories: the insane, those suffering from feeblemindedness as a result of senility, idiots defined as those unable to guard themselves against common danger, imbeciles defined as unable to earn a living, inebriates, the deaf, dumb or blind and epileptics. The Idiots Act of 1886 already dealt with severe cases of mental defect. What was significant about the Commission's recommendations was the introduction of a new category, 'the feebleminded', that is persons presumed to be suffering from mental defect but not of a severe nature. These were defined as persons 'who may be capable of earning a living under favourable circumstances but are incapable (a) of competing on equal terms with normal fellows; or (b) of managing themselves or their affairs with ordinary prudence.' To this category was added the 'moral imbecile' a person convicted of an offence upon whom 'punishment had little or no deterrent effect' and who consistently displayed 'immoral or vicious tendencies'. The Commission got no further than a recommendation for the Board of Control (established to supervise lunacy and idiot establishments) to supervise these and separate their care from the Poor Law and Prison administration.

Considerable agitation was already underway not only to extend State supervision of mental defectives but to create special powers for the indefinite detention of the feebleminded in institutions. The pressure came from organisations such as the National Association for the Welfare of the Feebleminded founded in 1896, the Eugenics Education Society, and the Charity Organisation Society founded in 1869. At a meeting of the National Association for the Feebleminded in 1909, the social objectives of these groups were spelt out. A Dr Savage regarded the remedy for national decline as 'the adoption of measures for the early detention of the "unfit" and the prevention of their propagation.' W.H. Dickenson MP 'combated the view that the feebleminded formed a harmless element in the community, for in that class existed a potentiality even for serious crime. At least they were a drag on progress.' A.F. Tredgold claimed, 'It was high time to stem the advancing tide of degeneracy. . . . Their propagation must be prevented.'[18]

Because of the delay by the government in implementing the provisions of the 1908 Commission on the Feebleminded, these organisations introduced their own bill into the House of Commons. The COS and the Eugenics Society initially introduced, independently of each other, Mental Defect bills into Parliament. Realising the futility of this they merged their efforts and in 1911 drew up a 'Feebleminded Persons (Control) Bill'.[19] This put the Board of Control (a body set up to oversee lunacy and idiot institutions) in control of a new category of persons, the 'feebleminded' previously not subject to any legislative or administrative control. It gave the Home Secretary the right to license existing homes and new ones for the reception of these. The categories of feebleminded listed in the bill were the senile, the defective found wandering, neglected or cruelly treated, those referred by the parent as in need of detention, or those transferred from special schools for the backward child, the parental home having been considered unsuitable to receive them. In addition it made knowingly marrying or abetting the marriage of a feebleminded person an offence. Two medical practitioners were required for certification.

In 1912, whilst this bill was being debated, the Government introduced their own measure, which in 1913 after considerable modification became the Mental Deficiency Act. It was amended by supporters of a mental deficiency act but, most of all, by its opponents. This measure was, initially, even more draconian than the previous one introduced to the House. It gave the Secretary of State power to detain those defectives charged with, though not convicted of, a crime, in a mental deficiency institution. This was later dropped, though the 1913 Act provided for the indefinite detention, subject to review, in mental deficiency institutions of 'moral imbeciles' usually referred from the courts. Second, it allowed detention of those defectives 'in whose case it is desirable in the interests of the community that they should be deprived of the opportunity of producing children'. Thirdly it allowed for detention on the grounds of 'other circumstances' specified solely by the Secretary of State — a very permissive power indeed. In the end the last two categories were dropped and those in the first bill retained plus an additional one. A woman considered feebleminded and in receipt of poor relief who was pregnant with or had given birth to an illegitimate child could be detained in a mental deficiency institution.[20]

It was assumed that this Act would lead to a sorting out of the mentally deficient from workhouses, the courts and other institutions, and their transfer to special institutions. It was also hoped that, gradually, the mass of mental defect in the community would be reduced due to the detention and therefore loss of procreative rights of the feebleminded. The Mental Deficiency bill was pursued on these grounds and it was accompanied by a very great deal of hysterical comment about the consequences of leaving the mentally deficient at large in the community. In 1913 when it looked as though the delaying tactics of its opponents would cause the government to drop the bill for want of parliamentary time, the Eugenics Education Society launched a counter-campaign against the critics of the bill. Their point of view was espoused by the Bishop of Down and Connor, Frederick D'Arcy, member of the Belfast Eugenics Society:

the essential point was the fact that members of the inefficient, feebleminded, subnormal class in the community were at present multiplying at a most enormous rate, whilst those of the effective class — the normal or the able — were increasing at a smaller rate. The meaning of that was that in a very short time — in a very few generations — all the abler stock would be wiped out of the community. That was a terrific fact and he thought that the public should be made aware of it. What they really wanted above all things, was to prevent the marriage of the unfit, and almost anything would be worth doing to that end. In some parts of America, he believed they were acting with great vigour in the matter, but in this country the people had not been awakened to the facts of the case. It was a sad thing, but it was true, that much of that charitable and social life was but aggravating the evil.[21]

Detention in institutions was very much on the agenda of social hygiene. Elizabeth Sloan Chesser recommended, in 1911, detention and a colony system for alcoholics, vagrants and the feebleminded as well as compulsory treatment for those suffering from sexually transmitted diseases which would have involved a similar power of detention.[22] In addition the desire to institutionalise was accompanied less and less by the rhetoric of rehabilitation. It was increasingly assumed that alcoholism, prostitution, vagrancy and to a large extent unemployment were a complex of problems with a single root — feeblemindedness. Since this was an innate and inherited condition, contemporary wisdom saw the institution as more important as a means of reproductive control than of rehabilitation.

Were these measures, as Havelock Ellis claimed, an extension of the great reforming impulses of the nineteenth century? The minority who led the parliamentary struggle in the House of Commons against these measures did not think so. This struggle was conducted chiefly by the Liberal MP for Stoke-on-Trent, Josiah Wedgwood. He is known for his opposition to the Mental Deficiency Bill of 1913 but he was also very hostile to a number of other measures which the Liberal Home Secretary, Reginald McKenna, introduced into the Commons between 1911 and 1915. These included the Criminal Law Amendment Act, better known as the White Slave Traffic Act, and the Inebriacy Bill. The Criminal Law Amendment Act provided extensive powers for the police to arrest someone suspected of procurement for prostitution. It also permitted flogging for conviction on a second offence. The Inebriacy Bill — which was eventually dropped — allowed the detention and compulsory treatment of drunks who had committed one offence or those who were repeatedly intoxicated.

Wedgwood saw these measures as running against the liberal tradition of freedom of the individual. Many of their proponents spoke rather disparagingly of him as having sacrificed social reform and social progress for this ideal. Was this altogether true? Wedgwood supported medical inspection of schoolchildren by the local authorities and he wanted more spent on state medical services for blind and deaf children. Frederick Handel Booth, MP, his ally in these matters, argued during the Criminal Law Amendment Debate that the extension of national insurance against unemployment to domestic servants would do more to combat prostitution than the harassment and arrest of procurers. Moreover Booth believed in better sex education for the young. 'I consider the real responsibility of the grave evils with which we are now faced arises in large measure from the ignorance of these youthful people, an ignorance which has been encouraged by the prudery of the older people.'[23] In addition, opposition to these measures came from the political wing of liberalism most committed to measures of social amelioration. Though not all new Liberals took this view, the *Nation*, newspaper of the new Liberalism, was a fervent opponent both of eugenics and the Mental Deficiency Bill.

Wedgwood and his allies were not therefore simple proponents of *laissez faire*. Wedgwood's reasons for opposing these measures were far more complex. His objection particularly to the Mental Deficiency Bill was not only that it was an infraction of rights but also that it was a class measure. In practice, the poor and unprotected would fall victim to it. Moreover, Wedgwood claimed, the assumption that this would be the case was widely accepted by those who framed and supported the bills. L.T. Hobhouse, the new Liberal, agreed. He was not against legislation in principle but he took exception to this particular measure,

> Even in the case of the feebleminded I feel strongly that some legislative provision is desirable but it would be provision in the interests of the feebleminded themselves, and not in the interests of eugenics, nor in the interests of a policy of which the real objective is to police the poorer classes.[24]

Wedgwood went further. He believed the Mental Deficiency Bill exemplified the attitude of mind which saw the working class solely in the light of their economic efficiency or inefficiency, as a 'wealth product or a drag', its objective being to separate the productive from the unproductive. Referring to a speech by Leslie Scott, later president of CAMW, he claimed,

> He viewed the child as a potential producer of wealth, as a citizen who is not only to be trained to look after himself but to be able to earn something as he grew up. I do not know whether he thinks that the only end of existence is to produce wealth for other people . . . The only interest of Hon. Members who support this Bill is the production of wealth by the community.[25]

Wedgwood's second objection was that the bill was brought about by 'artificial agitation':

> Last year we had a sudden, tearing agitation got up over what was called the 'White Slave Traffic' Bill. This House passed the Bill and

then discovered there was no trade at all. (Hon. Members 'oh no')
Not a single white slave trader has been unmasked since. . . . A similar
agitation has been got up now.[26]

There were, claimed Wedgwood, constant *ad hominem* arguments from
supporters of these measures, lists of illegitimate children born to
feebleminded women, the pedigrees of criminal families, the claims made
that babies would die if the measure was not passed. But this hysteria
was not justified. The problem of the white slaver and the mentally deficient was, Wedgwood felt, not a real problem but a problem got up in
the imagination and magnified by it.

Third, Wedgwood strongly objected to 'government by experts'. The
categories in the Mental Deficiency Bill were so vague that it left tremendous leeway to medical practitioners. They had, through the power of
certification granted to them by the Mental Deficiency Bill, been given
the authority of police and courts combined. In a later fight against an
amendment to the 1913 Mental Deficiency Act, in 1927, Wedgwood put
his objections in this way:

Now we get the usual amending Bill, giving a little more power to
the State, and to the experts, hemming in a little more closely those
who approach the borderline. . . . The expert has his own way with
the institution. He may lock the door or open the door. He can sentence
a person to imprisonment not for nine months but for life. The experts after all are so very often expert merely in the imagination of
others. My every reading of history fills me with horror at the thought
of priestly authority . . . that danger, that awful nightmare over
humanity has gradually vanished; let us take care lest in this generation we build up by their worship, by this prostration before the experts a new terror as horrible as the old.[27]

Finally Wedgwood associated this spate of legislative fervour with
the decline of liberalism as he had known it — not its political but its
moral decline. It had been transformed into something else, something
closer to conservatism and shed its old progressive and radical role in
British politics.

Was Wedgwood correct? There are alternative views of the historical
origins of the science of the body and the increasing importance of confinement.[28] In his volume on the *History of Sexuality*, Foucault treats
the development of the human sciences, and eugenics as arising from
the theoretical structure of science in its initial phase of observation and

classification. The application of this to the individual, led, so it is argued, to the rise of modern medical institutions and practices. In its train came a form of domination and power exercised over the body which worked by forcing the person to reveal themselves, to be observed and categorised in the name of science. Whilst it proclaimed itself, particularly in the area of sexuality, to be liberating — and here the name of Havelock Ellis crops up — it was, in fact, insidiously repressive. The willingness of social hygienists to bring sexual questions into the open, to categorise and record the sexual life was, in itself, destructive of privacy and freedom. Along with loss of privacy went an attempt on the part of social hygienists to direct and control sexuality. They did this not by prohibition but by the application of technique, particularly that of getting a patient into a situation of sympathetic collusion with the expert to whom he or she revealed their private thoughts. Thus the classic technique in Foucault's account of the human sciences is psycho-analysis.

Foucault's history writes in terms of 'the gaze', the revelation of social and family relationships, in all their intimate detail, through psycho-analysis, surveys and investigations, through in fact, the techniques of modern social and medical investigation. The impulse of self revelation and the treatment of the individual as an object of investigation, creates in people a sense of powerlessness and oppression. But this powerlessness and oppression is a phenomenon which transcends class:

> If one writes the history of sexuality in terms of repression, relating this repression to the utilisation of labour capacity, one must suppose that sexual controls were the more intense and meticulous as they were directed at the poorer classes; one has to assume that they followed the path of greatest domination and the most systematic exploitation, the young adult possessing nothing more than his life force, had to be the primary target of a subjugation destined to shift the energy available for useless pleasure towards compulsory labour. But this does not appear to be the way things actually happened. On the contrary, the most rigorous techniques were formed and more particularly applied first with the greatest intensity in the most privileged and politically dominant classes.[29]

Foucault does not deny the application of social hygiene to working class life. He sees this as occurring in France first as birth control in the eighteenth century, second with the moralisation of the working class family in the early nineteenth century and third in the stamping out of perversions in the late nineteenth century, a process which spread to all classes. What Foucault does deny is the ontological significance of class in the rise of social hygiene.

What is interesting about his analysis is the absence from it of any discussion of the differential birth rate. This was an obsessive concern of the British social hygiene movement well into the twentieth century. By the differential birth rate was meant not merely a general rise or fall in the population but the greater birth rate in the working classes compared to other social groups. The British eugenics and birth control movements were deeply concerned at the social implications of this and much of their efforts were directed at redressing it.

In contrast the demographic history of France followed a different course. France had a static or declining population throughout much of the nineteenth and twentieth centuries and a smaller industrial working class. It had, however, a large, non-industrial middle class. In this social situation, marriage alliances or mesalliances, delayed marriage and inheritance were all significant for the preservation of middle class income and status. The social management of the family in France might very well reflect this. It would lead, as Foucault claims, to an excessive concern with the social and sexual behaviour of the middle class adolescent. Clearly, there are aspects of British social hygiene which also reflect these preoccupations but it would be wrong to make these the nub of social hygiene in Britain.

Jacques Donzelot in his book *The Policing of Families* makes a number of more pertinent comments. Donzelot describes the process by which the family became subject to social management in the nineteenth and twentieth centuries.[30] This social management included the introduction into the family economy of welfare measures and family benefits plus the rise of the counselling system and of groups of experts and pedagogues who tendered advice to the family. He suggests that women and children — the discontented members of the old patriarchal family — invited in the experts to redress the balance of power in family relationships. Social hygiene became a weapon by which family relationships were prised apart and the moral and the economic power of the father reduced. The privacy and integrity of the family had been a shield for patriarchy but the growth of a science of child rearing and sexology and the multiplication of experts in these areas destroyed patriarchal authority. Small wonder then, that the advance guards of feminist thought and social hygiene were in alliance.

Or were they? The expert was not invited into the family by the women. He or she invited themself. Sometimes they forced themselves past the door. They were able to do so only in certain clearly defined situations. The privacy of the family to which Donzelot refers belonged to the era of the self sufficient economies of the peasant and artisan. Privacy went, not with a family quarrel, but with the growth of a wage earning proletariat. One of the first legislative disruptions of family relations in Britain appeared on the introduction of the Poor Law of 1834 when wives and husbands were received into the workhouse separately. Pauperisation and the arrival of the 'expert' occurred side by side. Similarly, the officials of the Charity Organisation Society used indigency as the key which opened the doors of the homes of the poor. On the application for relief, a scientific assessment of the needs of the family was made and visitation of the home followed. This led to advice, regulation of expenditure and other forms of interference. Even in the 1930s depression, it was the means test applied to applicants for relief, usually male heads of households, that led to intervention in the relationships of the family. The strictures about children's earnings counting as household income, applied under the means test, were a potent force in disrupting the internal politics of the family.

Many of the other intrusions of the expert into the family were equally uninvited. For example access to the family was frequently sought through the courts. The object of many social hygienists was to make those convicted of an offence subject to psychological examination. The eugenicist W.A. Potts pioneered this process, in what became known as the Birmingham system when he became official psychologist to the courts there.[31] Either way, the social hygienist did not wait to be invited. In addition, we have already looked briefly at the role of legislation in extending the power of social hygiene and the right to intervene in the family. This would be a surprising outcome of a purely feminine revolt against patriarchy.

On the contrary there is evidence of a subterranean revolt among families at the intrusion of the expert in which women took part equally with men. In 1956 the National Council for Civil Liberties brought a number of such cases referred to it before the Royal Commission on Mental Illness and Mental Deficiency. They included,

> Dorothy who when notice of her marriage reached the eyes of the authority . . . was seized at the door of the Register Office as she was entering to get married. We understand that she was forcibly conveyed to the institution van and carried off to the institution where she was detained for two years. She then, we believe, escaped and succeeded in contracting her marriage. To the best of our knowledge she has not been traced.[32]

There was also Elaine who had a

normal school education. Detained at the age of fifteen when doing normal work after conviction of mother by the Court. Transferred to institution with no resident medical staff and employed in a laundry operating electrical steam pressers at one shilling per week. Escaped to family, recaptured by the police, lodged in the cells overnight and returned to institution. Escaped a second time, was hidden by neighbours who told police they could prosecute if they liked but they were not going to hand back a perfectly normal girl. Neighbours then consulted a legal advice bureau who got the girl independently examined. Shown not to be mentally deficient and after much negotiation order was discharged in 1949. Girl immediately obtained normal factory work at £4 10s per week.[33]

More remarkable is the absence in Foucault and Donzelot of any discussion of eating. This, like sex, has an aesthetic side and is often conducted within the family and is symbolic of its relationships — as the institution of the British Sunday dinner shows. It was also the object of constant advice and admonition from the expert in this period. What Foucault sees as absent in connection with the sexuality of the working class male — the repression of libido — is certainly there in connection with eating. The advice tendered by nutritional experts shows the strong relationship between the repression of libido and the direction of energy into useful work. The discourse on eating was firmly built on the question of class, income and work. Scientific eating clearly demonstrates the role of social hygiene in constituting an efficient, wage earning producer.

To say this is not to deny the phenomenon Donzelot observes that the middle class mother increasingly had recourse to the expert or pedagogue on child rearing and psychological development in this period. It is to deny its ontological significance. The middle-class mother certainly saw the advice of the expert as one of the ways in which, in an age of white collar professional work, the family's educational capital and ability to reproduce its status and social acceptability could be safeguarded. However this was not the only way. The desire to maintain middle class status through the family was one important aspect of eugenics. But this could be done in more direct ways. Social hygiene for the middle classes was more likely to be sought in terms of relieving them of tax burdens, seeking tax allowances, graded by income, for children and helping with private educational expenses. These measures were the staple of much of the Eugenics Society's work in the 1920s. It hoped thereby to deflect the middle class from what it considered to be the socially disastrous expedient of protecting their income by limiting their families.

Was Wedgwood therefore correct in his estimation of the role of social hygiene? First was it a measure directed at the poor? Both its supporters and critics suggested that it was. Behind the agitation for the Mental Deficiency Bill was a strong, insistent theme about the economic cost of feeblemindedness. As one commentator put it in 1912, the hope of reducing the poor rate would do more for the progress of the Mental Deficiency Bill than knowledge of the laws of Mendelian genetics.[34] The figure of £20 million expended on poor relief was frequently bandied about. Whilst poor relief would not disappear as a charge on the community because of mental deficiency policy, it was argued that the latter could aid its reduction. This belief existed because of the identification of the feebleminded with the residuum — that section of the unemployable and unemployed much discussed in Edwardian economic thought. Bishop D'Arcy described them in these terms,

> Again there is the respectable married pauper whose 'home' is the workhouse, in which his wife is confined of a large family, who got out of the workhouse so long as begging is profitable and no longer. . . . The workhouse clothes are cast off, the rags resumed and the wandering mother and children, arrayed in all the paraphernalia of beggardom go upon another journey of pillage and vagrancy only to seek again the sheltering walls of the State-supported institution when begging does not pay any longer. I have known many families brought up under these conditions and the ratepayers of today and tomorrow will continue to groan and sweat under the yolk of taxation for the care and support of the degenerates so long as this State aided lunacy and pauper manufactory receives from the State and the ratepayers such solid financial and moral support.[35]

Elizabeth Sloan Chesser believed that the chief cause of pauperism was not lack of money but 'ignorance, indifference, inherited slovenliness and improvidence'. Chesser cited several examples of this including the bad management of the household wage and lack of nutritional knowledge. This could be counteracted by instruction in domestic management. But she went further. To this she added the eugenic control of heredity, including the sterilisation of the feebleminded, compulsory medical treatment, and a ban on the marriage of 'degenerates'.

With these measures she believed 'so-called "poverty" could be reduced by 80 per cent'.[36]

Social hygiene was offered as an alternative or supplement to poor relief, insurance and other means for relieving poverty. Therefore when E.J. Lidbetter began in 1910 to compile a list of pauper pedigrees for the Eugenics Education Society — a task which lasted throughout the 1920s — it was to show that, contrary to the assumption of the Royal Commission on the Poor Law (1909), unemployment was caused by poor physical and mental heredity. The implication of this was that it could be controlled by the management of heredity.[37] In 1934 Havelock Ellis returned to this point. An ultimate goal of social hygiene was reducing and controlling the unemployable and unemployed in the working class by means other than charity or social insurance, by, in fact, regulation of sexuality.

> Our society . . . recognizes a certain responsibility for its members. And if it is responsible for maintaining them when once brought into the world that means it must assume control for bringing them in. Society cannot accept responsibility for those of its members whose existence in the world it has not sanctioned. We profess the contrary, we put up a fine bluff. But we know, at heart, that this is the core of the situation. Meanwhile we keep alive the unemployed remnants of the great proletarian armies of old. We either put them on the dole or we exercise charity. For in one country they like to feel they have a legal right to a dinner and, in another country, they like to regard it as a gracious gift. Indirectly in one way or another, in the end they will both have to pay for it.[38]

Notes

1. See *Journal of Hygiene*, 1910-30, vols. 10-30.
2. Report of the Committee on Physical Deterioration, 1904.
3. J.A. Thomson, 'Biology and Social Hygiene', *Quarterly Review*, vol. 246 (1926) pp. 28-48.
4. J. Huxley, 'The Applied Science of the Next Hundred Years', *Life and Letters*, vol. 11 (October 1934), p. 40.
5. Havelock Ellis, *The Task of Social Hygiene* (Constable and Co., London, 1912).
6. Elizabeth Sloan Chesser, 'The Health of the Nation' *The National Review*, vol. 56 (1911) p. 755.
7. See G.R. Searle, *The Quest for National Efficiency* (Blackwell, Oxford, 1971), and *Eugenics and Politics in Britain, 1900-14* (Noordhof International, Leyden, 1976); D. MacKenzie, *Statistics in Britain 1865-1930* (Edinburgh University Press, Edinburgh, 1981). Lyndsay A. Farrall, *The Origins and Growth of the English Eugenics Movement*,

1865-1925, unpublished PhD thesis, University of Indiana, 1970.

8. *The Times*, 25 July 1912.

9. See S. Neville Rolfe, 'Autobiographical Notes' in *Social Biology and Welfare* (Allen and Unwin, London, 1949) and Joan Austoker, *Biological Education and Social Reform, the BSHC, 1925-42*, unpublished MA thesis, University of London, 1981.

10. See Annual Reports of the CAMW 1920-39.

11. See NIIP Papers, LSE, and H.J. Welch and C.S. Myers, *Ten Years of Industrial Psychology* (Sir Isaac Pitman and Sons, London, 1932).

12. See the report of the founding of the National Council on the 4 May 1922 in the *Journal of Mental Science*, vol. 68 (July 1922), pp. 278-81.

13. Olga Nethersole, *The Inception of the League* (People's League of Health, London, 1920), p. 2.

14. See W.E. Tanner, *Sir William Arbuthnot Lane* (Ballière, Tindall and Co., London, 1946), p. 128.

15. S. Henning Belfrage, *What's Best to Eat* (Heinemann, London, 1926), p. 6 (dedicated to Sir William Arbuthnot Lane).

16. See P. Weiler, *The New Liberalism* (Garland, New York, 1982), pp. 90-1; José Harris, *William Beveridge, A Biography* (Oxford University Press, Oxford, 1977).

17. Report of the Royal Commission on the Feebleminded, *BMJ*, 8 August, 1908, p. 329. See also Gillian Sutherland, *Ability, Merit and Measurement, Mental Testing and English Education, 1880-1940* (Oxford University Press, Oxford, 1984).

18. 'National Association for the Feebleminded', *BMJ*, 22 May, 1909, pp. 1243-4.

19. For details of the Eugenics Society Bill, see *BMJ*, 2 December, 1911, p. 1497. (The bill was first presented 15 April 1912, Second Reading 17 May 1912).

20. 'The Mental Deficiency Bill', *BMJ*, 25 May 1912, pp. 1193-4.

21. 'Frederick D'Arcy, Bishop of Down and Connor', *The Northern Whig*, 12 February 1914.

22. Chesser, 'The Health of the Nation', *National Review*, vol. 56 (1911), pp. 755-62.

23. Booth, H of C Deb, 22 April 1912, vol. 39, p. 580.

24. Wedgwood Papers, Keele University, Hobhouse to Wedgwood, 5 December 1912.

25. Wedgwood, ibid., H of C Deb, 28 May 1913, vol. 53, pp. 243-4.

26. Ibid.

27. Wedgwood, H of C Deb, 18 March 1927, vol. 203, pp. 2336-7 (Quoted in MH51/565).

28. M. Foucault, *History of Sexuality*, vol. 1 (Pantheon, New York, 1978). For Britain see David Armstrong, *The Political Anatomy of the Body* (Cambridge University Press, Cambridge, 1983).

29. Foucault, ibid., p. 120.

30. J. Donzelot, *The Policing of Families* (Pantheon, New York, 1979).

31. See W.A. Potts, 'Crime and Delinquency', *The People's League of Health Lectures* (Routledge and Sons, London, 1926).

32. National Council for Civil Liberties. Minutes of Evidence to the Royal Commission on the Law Relating to Mental Illness and Mental Deficiency, 1956-7, HMSO, Cmnd 169, p. 1135.

33. NCCL, ibid., p. 1139.

34. Richard Leeper, Discussion at the Royal Academy of Medicine in Ireland (Section of State Medicine) 19 January 1912. Reported in the *Dublin Journal of Medicine*, vol. 123, (1912), p. 294.

35. Richard Leeper, 'A Note on the Causation of Insanity in Ireland', *Dublin Journal of Medicine*, vol. 123 (1912), p. 184.

36. Elizabeth Sloan Chesser, 'The Lancashire Operative', *The National Review*, vol. 54 (1909), p. 690.

37. Report of the Committee on Poor Law Reform, *Eugenics Review*, vol. 2 (1910), pp. 167-94.

38. Havelock Ellis, *My Confessional* (John Lane, The Bodley Head, London, 1934), p. 23.

3 A DYNASTY OF EXPERTS

> I have a rigid distrust of experts, and I hesitate to subscribe to a recommendation made solely on the advice of experts — a recommendation which if adopted would go far in my opinion towards the setting up of a medical dynasty in this country.
>
> (George Gibson (Mental Hospital and Institutional Workers' Union) *TUC Reports*, 1934, p. 399.)

Social hygienists covered pretty well the whole social spectrum except, significantly, the majority of the Labour movement. The membership of social hygiene groups reveals two significant things. First there is a high degree of overlap and interconnection. Second, social hygiene laid down roots very deep into the British social and political system.

We shall begin with an important and influential family, the Cecils. The Cecils are an aristocratic, landed family, deeply involved with the Conservative Party, and having extensive connections with other aristocratic families. They were involved with the social hygiene movement in the first three decades of the twentieth century. Arthur Balfour, a British Conservative Prime Minister, was a Cecil through his mother (a daughter of the Marquess of Salisbury). His sister, Eleanor, married the philosopher and political economist Henry Sidgwick. Balfour was present and made a speech at the International Eugenics Congress held in 1912 and became an honorary vice president of the Eugenics Society in 1913. He voted for the Mental Deficiency Bill in 1913 and later became president of the CAMW. Eleanor Sidgwick was also a supporter of the 1913 Bill. Evelyn Cecil, Balfour's brother-in-law, was one of the group of Members of Parliament who pressed the government in the Commons about the progress of the Mental Deficiency Bill thereby hoping to facilitate its passage. The third son of the Marquess of Salisbury, Edgar Algernon Cecil known as Robert, Conservative MP for East Marylebone, was credited by Wedgwood with doubts about the 1913 Act. He was certainly more liberal politically than others of his family. However, he became a vice president of the CAMW formed to put into effect the provisions of the 1913 Act. The second son, Lord William Gascoyne Cecil was Bishop of Exeter from 1913 to 1936. He was one of the petitioners in 1929 who asked the government to introduce voluntary sterilisation of the mentally deficient.[1]

The old traditional landed elite were prominent in pushing for the

1913 bill. Lord Claud Hamilton, son of the Duke of Abercorn, whose mother was a relation of the Duke of Bedford, worked in Parliament for the bill. Lord Richard Cavendish (Duke of Devonshire's family) was part of the COS deputation to the government in 1913 which pressed for action on mental deficiency. Others on that deputation included Arthur Annesley, Lord Valentia, premier baronet of Ireland and owner of 7,000 acres, Reginald Brabazon, Earl of Meath representing the National Association for the Feebleminded and Constance Shaftesbury, daughter of the Earl of Grosvenor.[2]

Even in 1937 the Eugenics Society could boast among its numbers the seventh Earl of Beauchamp who was married to the sister of the second Duke of Westminster and owned 5,000 acres and the Earl of Iveagh (the Guinness family) who married into the Earl of Onslow's family. Walter Guinness, before he became Lord Iveagh, represented Southend as a Unionist from 1912 to 1927 and voted for the 1913 Bill. In addition the Earl and Countess of Limerick were members. So were the Honorable Marcus Pelham, from the family of the Earls of Chichester and Yarborough, and the Countess of Dartmouth.[3]

Social hygiene was not therefore devoid of aristocrats but was it aristocratic? Its links with voluntary charity inevitably drew many prominent leaders of society into it as patrons. The People's League specialised, in particular, in putting on fund-raising events which were part of the London social season. It was said of Lady St. Helier of the CAMW that she was 'indefatigable in service of the poor and, in society, famed for her brilliant art of entertaining!'[4] But were these aristocratic patrons any more than figureheads?

Wedgwood suspected that social hygiene represented a convergence of interests between the political parties and that some deeper social purpose was being served by it. Social hygiene certainly united figures across party and social background and it did so because it was created to stem a threat usually called 'the rising tide of degeneracy'. This was a threat which challenged or was assumed to challenge a whole series of institutions — Empire, the family, the ratepayer, morals, national fitness and ultimately social stability. So long as social hygiene offered a remedy for these kinds of ills it transcended narrow political and social differences.

An important stimulus to aristocratic participation came from the Empire. The Cecils were well known for their involvement with Imperial concerns. The Earl of Meath, Reginald Brabazon, was the first president of the British College of Physical Education, the Lads' Drill Association and the Duty and Discipline Movement. He was the instigator of Empire Day an annual celebration of Imperial Glory in British schools.[5] The Earl of Iveagh and his wife were 'enthusiastic supporters of Imperialist ideals'[6] and involved in projects for Canadian emigration. The social round, a sense of public duty, the new fad of Empire and national efficiency could all be said to have drawn a section of the aristocracy into social hygiene.

Another interest which may have had this effect was the land. Martin Wiener has, in a recent book, noted the nostalgia for Britain's rural past which accompanied the industrialisation and urbanisation of the nineteenth and twentieth centuries[7]. This nostalgia was influential in the social hygiene movement. Leslie Scott (later Lord Chief Justice Scott) is a case in point. He was a prominent parliamentary supporter of the 1913 Act whilst a Conservative MP (1910-29), a member of the National Association for the Feebleminded, CAMW and the Eugenics Society. As well as social hygiene, Scott was 'interested in all questions of social and industrial reform particularly in connection with the development of agriculture and the improvement of the conditions of life affecting the rural population'.[8] He served on the Council for the Preservation of Rural England of which he was a founder member and was President of the National Association of Parish Councils, a bastion of English rural life. Charles Bathurst, active in the Campaign for the Mental Deficiency Bill of 1913, was also the founder in 1907 of the Central Land Association.[9] The Marchioness of Aberdeen and Temair, Vice President of the People's League of Health was an advocate of town and country planning and the smallholding movement.[10]

The traditional social authority of aristocratic England was in the country. So, along with the suburbs, was the major electoral strength of the Conservative Party. But to describe this interest in land as traditionalist would be misleading. Tradition in British agriculture, in the sense of a peasantry and ancient methods of cultivation, had disappeared in the preceding centuries, except for Ireland and parts of Scotland and Wales. With these exceptions, British agriculture, whatever the social continuity represented by the landed families over the centuries, was capitalist, scientific and innovatory. Moreover the old traditional land-owning classes were leavened by members from different social origins. Viscount Burnham (Harry Lawson), a member of the CAMW, owned 6000 acres. His title derived from 1919 and his social position from being, until 1928, Managing Proprietor of the *Daily Telegraph*. He was involved successively whilst a Unionist MP (1910-16) with the 1913 Act, the CAMW and the People's League of Health.[11]

It was not nostalgia for a way of life which had passed away for ever that prompted interest in things rural but the need to deal with urgent contemporary problems. First among these was the desire to stem the physical and social degeneration brought about by city life. Much importance was attributed, in this connection, to the town and country planning movement and the provision of open spaces for the urban dweller. This was considered to have a beneficial effect upon the health and the morals of the working class. J.A. Thomson had listed 'place' as one of the three aspects of social hygiene and his friend and collaborator Patrick Geddes was deeply involved in the movement for urban regeneration. In addition the political platform of Conservative groups, hoping to attract working class votes, offered suburbanisation, by means of better transport between home and work and the provision of smallholdings, as a programme of social reform.[12] Schemes for resettlement of the poor on the land were popular in both parties but they had a particular appeal to the Liberals for whom the country smallholder was the bulwark of rural political support in Wales and the West. Liberals hoped that the spread of smallholdings would act as an ideological barrier to the growth of socialism. They also saw resettlement on the land as a cure for industrial unemployment. Hence Asquith's patronage of Arbuthnot Lane's health programme which included the resettlement of the urban unemployed on the land.

There were other connections with social hygiene. A strong element in eugenics was predisposed to the rural. R.A. Fisher, the geneticist and Eugenics Society secretary, linked urbanisation to racial decay. Urbanisation had made 'money' not fitness the criterion of social success whereas early rural and semi-tribal societies had measured success by bravery, leadership, and the agrarian and domestic virtues. It had also rewarded philoprogenitiveness whereas modern society rewarded infertility.[13] The city was, according to Fisher, the enemy of the natural aristocrat, a view shared by W.C.D. Whetham, historian of science, agricultural expert and eugenicist. They saw in eugenics a means of retrieving what had been lost in urbanisation.[14]

Sir Arbuthnot Lane of the New Health Society carried this even further. His views on the effect of city life on heredity were similar to Fisher's. In addition he believed urbanisation had led to a deterioration in the city dwellers' diet. Urbanisation had increased the distance between the supply of food and the market and led to the use of additives in food, the processing and preservation of food and to a bland and monotonous diet from whose consumption most of modern health problems derived. Arbuthnot Lane therefore led campaigns for food purity, and he hoped to rescue men and women from bad food by sending them to the country to grow their own. This would have another effect. It would remove the individual from the nervous tension and debility brought on by city life. It would also, he believed, cure industrial unemployment.[15]

There was wide support for social hygiene among the churches. This was an era in which eugenicists pronounced upon moral questions and churchmen became eugenicists. Claud Montefiore was a leading theologian of reformed Judaism and a member of the Eugenics Society. He was signatory to the letters to *The Times* in support of the Mental Deficiency Bill in 1912 and of a later petition to the government in 1929 asking for voluntary sterilisation of the mentally deficient.[16] Edward Bristow has recently noted his involvement with the campaign against white slavery in this period.[17] Among the free churches, the Baptist Union came out in favour of sterilisation in March 1935. W.B. Selbie, Principal of Mansfield College, Oxford, and a Congregationalist, and J. Scott Lidgett, editor of *The Methodist Times*, 1907-18, were both in favour of the 1913 Mental Deficiency Act.[18] The Church of England was considered by the Eugenics Society to be particularly favourable to its cause. In 1910, Mrs Pinsent, a member of the Royal Commission on the Feebleminded and also of the Eugenics Society, read a paper before the Church Congress at Cambridge on the subject of the multiplication of the unfit. It was very well received.[19] W.C.D. Whetham commended the Church of England for its enlightened attitude to eugenics in the *Eugenics Review* of 1910.[20] Two years later the Convocation of the Church of England passed a resolution in support of the Mental Deficiency Bill. Cosmo Lang, Archbishop of York, Randall Davidson, Archbishop of Canterbury, the Bishops of Wakefield, Manchester and Chester wrote to the papers in its support. In 1929, the signatories to the Grand National Council of Citizens' Unions' petition in favour of sterilisation included the Bishops of Exeter, Kingston and Durham.[21]

Some of these Church of England bishops were politically Conservative. During the 1920s and 1930s the Very Reverend W.R. Inge, Dean of St Paul's, became famous or notorious for his broadcasts and public statements on eugenics. They were so socially conservative that they embarrassed the younger members of the Eugenics Society.[22] Similarly, Hensley Henson, Bishop of Durham, an advocate of sterilisation, was famous for his defence of the established order, 'his outspoken opposition to Socialist remedies often aroused irritation and even hostility among the miners in Durham and the surrounding areas.'[23] These churchmen were also characterised by the modernism of their theology. Inge, along with the Bishop of Exeter and Frederick D'Arcy, Bishop of Down and Connor, all published books in the tradition of liberal protestantism attempting to show that science and religion were compatible.[24] In particular they tried to reconcile evolutionary biology with Christianity. Bishop Barnes of Birmingham, for example, a eugenicist and supporter of sterilisation carried this scientific spirit in theology as far as ecclesiastical authority would allow. In the 1920s, he was reprimanded by his superiors for his famous 'gorilla sermons'[25] in which he traced the hand of God in Darwinian evolution. Barnes's reputation as an outspoken modernist and his speeches on the rights of the decent English working man — which will be described below — earned him the approval of Ramsay MacDonald who made him Bishop of Birmingham during the first Labour Government in 1924.

Their views on evolution may have predisposed these churchmen to a more 'Darwinian' view of social questions. Frederick D'Arcy, Bishop of Down and Connor exemplifies this. An Irish protestant bishop he was a signatory to the Ulster Covenant in 1913. D'Arcy wrote several essays reconciling evolution with Christian dogma. He also had strong views on social questions. He was president of the Belfast Branch of the Eugenics Education Society formed in 1911 to get the Mental Deficiency Bill extended to Ireland. He saw mental deficiency policy as a means by which the 'honest' working man could be protected against the competition of the feckless and incompetent. In 1912, he wrote

> The unskilled worker or the worker whose capacity is such that he cannot take his place as a recognized member of any trade or form of employment, became too often an outcast from the camp of workers and has no protection against the force of competition which drives him downwards. Thus, we have an unemployed and unemployables; and among the very feeblest classes of the community this most terrible result, that pay is lowest and competition keenest and the burden of supporting the poor falls upon the very poor. Nor do the ordinary efforts of the benevolent help these outcasts relieve the poorest of this burden; for the simple and badly paid employments in which alone the neediest can earn a living are taken by the labour home and the charitable institution as the means by which the tramp may be rescued from his misery and the poorest workers find themselves competing with subsidized labour.[26]

D'Arcy saw mental deficiency policy as the means to control the residuum of the unemployable. He believed this offered a genuine measure of social amelioration to the industrial worker. He wrote in this fashion for the paper, *The Empire Citizen*, in the 1920s.[27] This paper was a descendant of the pre-war social Imperialist tariff reform newspapers aimed at the working man. It preached patriotism and the abandonment of the class war.

Bishop Barnes had similar views. He had a more anti-capitalist rhetoric — 'Modern England has no tyrant like the industrial magnate in whose work people enjoy no security of tenure and often work for a bare sustenance whilst he makes a fortune.'[28] On the other hand, he supported sterilisation for the same reasons that D'Arcy wanted mental defectives institutionalised. By removing the 'social derelicts' the respectable lower middle class and artisans would be relieved of an economic burden.

The Catholic Church in contrast was hostile to features of social hygiene, particularly birth control and sterilisation. Their opposition to eugenics surfaced after the Papal Bull of 1929 condemned it. However, even among Catholics, some of the other less controversial aspects of social hygiene won approval. In Ireland, Dr M.J. Nolan, resident medical superintendent of Down District Asylum and a Catholic, was one of the strongest opponents of proposals for sterilisation which were discussed during the campaign to get the Mental Deficiency Bill extended to Ireland. None the less, Nolan in 1906 suggested that consanguinous marriages and marriages of the mentally unfit should be prohibited, the state regulation of prostitution, temperance laws and registration of the mentally unsound.[29]

The most virulent opponents of social hygiene among Catholics tended to be those who had populist or radical social views. Thus it was *Eyewitness*, the newspaper edited by Cecil Chesterton and expressing a variety of Catholic radicalism, which ran the toughest campaign against the 1913 Mental Deficiency Bill.[30] Similarly the Distributivist League set up to propagate G.K. Chesterton's views on the need for radical economic reform worked hardest in the 1920s to persuade the Government against sterilisation although their views, if they had any weight at all with the Ministry of Health, had less than the opinions of the Catholic hierarchy.[31] G.K. Chesterton and Hilaire Belloc believed an intimate connection existed between capitalism and eugenics. It was the 'powerlessness' of the modern proletariat that allowed state intervention, bureaucratic control and the rearrangement of family life to take place. Thus, in a way strangely reminiscent of Donzelot, they saw the gospel of eugenics advancing as a propertyless working class dependent on wage labour emerged. Hence their desire to recreate in England an independent peasantry and artisanate, social groups which they also associated with the historical periods of Catholic dominance.

But were there, in fact, any capitalist eugenicists? One who undoubtedly fell into this category was Alfred Mond. He was a financial patron to the People's League and the New Health Society. Mond (1868-1930), was the son of a Jewish immigrant. Together with his partner, Sir John Brunner he founded Imperial Chemical Industries (ICI). Mond became the first Baron Melchett and played a considerable role in British political life. He was a Liberal MP before 1914, then Minister of Health in the Coalition Government of 1921-22. In 1926 he switched his allegiance to the Conservatives because of his conversion from free trade to Imperial protection.[32] Imperial Chemical Industries (ICI) was a large, monopolistic, technologically advanced and successful industry. In the 1920s, it was the model of a 'rationalised' industry. Rationalisation meant a movement towards monopoly in industry usually by the mutual agreement of a number of competing firms to plan production and marketing jointly. The next step was often merger. Rationalisation was particularly appropriate for industries like chemicals which required heavy investment in technological development. It was advocated, unsuccessfully, in the 1930s for the textile industry which was considered to over-produce from too many small and inefficient units. The solution suggested was to rationalise by a mutual agreement in the industry and to cut back production by closing certain plants. If successful, rationalisation could produce firms with great power and resources, like ICI. Mond, because of ICI's success, believed that rationalisation was the key to Britain's industrial problems 'only through more closely knit industrial entities, welding into one body, existing competitive industries, can British goods enlarge their world markets . . . by union still greater efficiency could be obtained . . .'.[33]

Mond was also deeply interested in social questions. In 1927, after the failure of the General Strike of 1926, with other leading industrialists and a number of trade union leaders, he inaugurated the Mond-Turner talks. These were intended to usher in an era of industrial peace by setting up joint negotiating bodies between the two sides of industry. The twin ideas of rationalisation and industrial cooperation were to have a great deal of influence upon the notion of what constituted scientific 'planning' in inter-war Britain.[34] Mond's interests also included social hygiene. Both he and Sir John Brunner were active supporters of the 1913 Mental Deficiency Bill. Robert Mond, Alfred's brother was on the executive of the Eugenics Education Society at the time.[35] Lord Melchett, as Alfred Mond became, and his wife Violet were signatories to a letter sent to the Ministry of Health in 1929 asking for voluntary sterilisation of the mentally deficient.[36]

Mond was strongly anti-socialist, but he believed the best defence against socialism was 'a contented, industrious and happy working class,' which would 'lend no ear to the leaders of the Third International at Moscow.'[37] This could be achieved by cooperation between the two sides of industry and by economic policy. In 1926 Mond was in favour of reflating the economy and of schemes for increasing employment. Social hygiene appealed to him for various reasons. First, it would raise the average level of fitness of the industrial worker. The proponents of rationalisation believed that improved health and vocational selection were the means to achieve a more efficient labour force and that this was as much a part of rationalisation as amalgamation of firms and reorganisation at the top. Rationalisation also meant negative eugenics. In 1931, the *Weekend Review*, an advocate of Mondism in industry, stated that industrial planning, 'must obey the biological principle of stimulating the fittest, the young and those capable of effort, as against the present dysgenic policy of overburdening them with the load of the elderly, the inefficient and the unemployables of all classes.'[38]

There were other industrialists involved in social hygiene. Lord Aberconway, Chairman of John Brown Shipbuilders, and a participant in the Mond-Turner talks, was a patron of the People's League as was Lord Leverhulme of Lever Brothers, a soap manufacturing firm. The Cadbury and Rowntree families, chocolate manufacturers and Quakers, with a traditional interest in social questions were deeply involved in social hygiene. The Cadburys were members of the Eugenics Society and the NIIP. B. Seebohm Rowntree, Chairman of Rowntree and Co. was ubiquitous in the 1920s and 1930s.[39] He was a member of NIIP and on nearly all the planning groups of the 1930s. W.H. Hazell of Hazell, Watson and Viney, Printers, was Treasurer of the Eugenics Society until his death in 1929, a member of the NIIP and a participant in the Mond-Turner talks.[40] In his will he left the Eugenics Society a legacy of £1000.[41]

These instances illustrate a general point about British society. There was a fluidity at the top of the social scale which reflects the integration between types of social status and wealth. From 1924 until his death in 1930, Arthur Balfour was president of the NIIP as well as the CAMW. He represented one thread of British social life with his connection with both the intellectual and the landed aristocracy. He was replaced by Lord D'Abernon, an aristocrat but also a coal owner who was deeply involved in industrial questions. Both the first Baron Melchett, Alfred Mond, and the second, Henry Mond, were members of the NIIP, the latter serving on the council of the NIIP in the 1930s. The Monds were a true example of entrepreneurial success. They had risen from relatively obscure social origins but they mixed on the council of the NIIP with Lord Dudley, just as Dame Lucy Houston, the millionairess daughter of a London warehouseman, mixed with the Marchioness of Aberdeen and Temair in the People's League. Wealth, industrial power, a career of public service, or prominent medical career and especially newspaper power brought elevation to the baronetcy and access to social elites. Even if social gradations were still observed and occasionally the cause of social embarrassment, there was little fundamental ideological or political disunity.

Social hygiene helped bind these groups together. In the pursuit of social hygiene, Conservatives cooperated with liberals, free traders with tariff reformers and pro-Home Rulers with Imperialists. It was not a divisive philosophy. When the question of land came up it was not in such a way as to question the social pre-eminence of the old landed elite. Land distribution and rural values were talked of as a means to civilise the proletariat. Therefore, Alfred Mond, the industrialist, and Herbert Henry Asquith, the Liberal Prime Minister and son of a small scale woollen manufacturer both felt at home in the ranks of the New Health Society, a group which advocated ruralisation.

The social hygiene movement drew into its orbit a considerable number of scientists. But it would be wrong to think of social hygiene originating as a movement to advance the professional interests of the scientific community. It may have served that function later but much of the original impetus came from outside the ranks of science. For example, interest in mentally deficient children was stimulated by the growth of public education in the late nineteenth century. Concern about those unable to keep up in class led to the Elementary Education Act (Blind and Deaf Children) in 1893 and the Education (Defective and Epileptic Children) Act 1899. Prior to the 1899 Act the provision of special educational facilities for the scholastically backward child was left to individual local authorities and, in the 1890s, only London County Council and Leicester provided these.

The need to cater for educationally backward children does not, however, explain why in the 1890s the feebleminded as a group should rouse such concern. This concern did not originate solely in the medical profession. George Shuttleworth, for example, medical superintendent of the Royal Albert Asylum for Idiots and Imbeciles in

Lancaster, helped frame an Act of Parliament which provided for the severely mentally retarded to be received into homes certified by the state. This was the Idiots Act of 1886. Shuttleworth was later involved in the campaign for the Mental Deficiency Bill and in the CAMW. However, in his textbook *Mentally Deficient Children* (1895) his views about the institutionalisation of the feebleminded were very different from those expressed in that campaign. In 1895 he believed the dangers of hereditary transmission of mental defect to be insignificant, that marriage between the feebleminded was rare and, on the occasions when it took place, harmless.

It is remarkable that of near a 1000 discharged patients who had passed under observation the two just mentioned are the only instances in which we have known marriages occur. It has indeed been urged as an objection to educating mentally deficient children and fitting them for work in the world that they would be thereby encouraged to marry and in consequence there would be a risk of multiplying mental defect in the progeny. Our experience lends no support to this view.[42]

The panic about the hereditary transmission of feeblemindedness, its social effects and the need for permanent institutionalisation came largely from outside the medical profession. The *BMJ* commented on this fact, when it referred, in 1898, to a recent meeting of the National Association for Promoting the Welfare of the Feebleminded. This meeting, it said 'is one more evidence of the widespread interest now taken in the feebleminded class and we are inclined to think that there is not now so much fear of the claims of this class being overlooked as of zeal occasionally outrunning knowledge.'[43]

The work of rousing interest in this subject was done by voluntary charitable bodies most of whose members were not medically qualified. The COS was one of the first groups to take an interest in feeblemindedness. In 1890 it set up a committee to investigate 50,000 school-children for defects of all kinds including mental deficiency.[44] In 1896 the National Association for Promoting the Welfare of the Feebleminded was founded. Its membership closely overlapped that of the COS. In 1898, Mary Dendy founded the Lancashire and Cheshire Society for the Permanent Care of the Feebleminded. Dendy's organisation was particularly fond of recommending institutionalisation. These groups exercised considerable influence over the report and recommendations of the Royal Commission on the Feebleminded (1908). The recommendations of the Royal Commission in 1908 were almost identical to those voted in 1904 at a conference of the National Association for the Feebleminded.[45] The deputation sent to the Home Secretary in 1910 asking for action to get the Mental Deficiency Bill through Parliament was composed of a mixture of officials from the COS, National Association for the Feebleminded and Eugenics Society. It was introduced by Sir Thomas Acland and included Sir William Chance, a barrister and vice president of the London COS. Chance was an expert on social problems, strongly anti-socialist and a defender of the old Poor Law.[46] The deputation also included Lady Frederick Cavendish, the Hon. Maude Stanley founder of the London Girls' Clubs, Lady Frederick Brudenell Bruce, the Earl of Meath, Mr William Bund, a barrister and chairman of Worcestershire Quarter Sessions, Ellen F. Pinsent, a member of Birmingham City Council, and Sir Edward Brabrook, a lawyer, anthropologist and folklore expert who was also interested in social problems.[47]

There were six medical people present. The characters of these show the degree to which a class of specialists in social hygiene was being created by the furore over the feebleminded. Among the six was Shuttleworth. The others included Dr Ettie Sayer, A.F. Tredgold and May Dickenson Berry. These three were employed by the London County Council. Tredgold from 1899 to 1901 was on a research scholarship funded by the LCC to survey the numbers of mentally deficient in the schools. Berry was an assistant Medical Officer of Health attached to the LCC education department. So was Ettie Sayer who was also consulting physician to the National Association for the Feebleminded. Harold Chapple MD and David Ferrier who were present were independent medical practitioners. Harold Chapple later married Sir William Arbuthnot Lane's daughter, Irene, and became involved in the New Health Society.

Apart from the National Council for Mental Hygiene none of the bodies described as social hygienist was formed purely of professionals. Of course it was perfectly possible to pursue professional interests in organisations composed of a mixture of lay and professional people. In particular, the psychologists promoting mental testing were ubiquitous and this probably reflects a degree of professional uncertainty and a desire to proselytise. Moreover, the opportunity to advance the cause of science was seized when it appeared. In 1913 *The Times*, during the debate in its letters columns over mental deficiency, received a letter from 31 prominent medical and scientific men asking for public support for research into the causes of feeblemindedness. The signatories to this included Sir William Osler, Clifford Allbutt, J.S. Haldane, C.S. Myers, C.S.

Sherrington, Sir Isambard Owen and Arthur Keith.

There were roughly two areas from which scientists or medical people were recruited into social hygiene, leaving aside individuals like Havelock Ellis, Thomson and Chesser who were self conscious ideologues of social hygiene. One was from medically qualified people involved in institutions and local government. These included the MOHs, particularly concerned with school medical inspections, the medical officers in prisons, workhouses, inebriacy institutions and poor relief committees. None the less, these were by no means wholly won over to social hygiene. In the Royal Commission of 1908 there was a small minority who opposed the prevailing opinion about institutionalisation and the inheritance of mental defect. Moreover, Arthur Newsholme (1857-1943) chief MOH for the Local Government Board 1908-19 kept up a barrage of criticism against the eugenic influence in public health. Although Newsholme was a critic of 'indiscriminate' charity he was also an environmental ameliorist.[48] If we examine the *Journal of Hygiene* for 1910-30, discussion is centred on questions of pure milk, contagious disease and mortality statistics. Some articles with eugenic inspiration begin to creep in but, on the whole, the practical day to day concerns of public health officers precluded them from totally embracing hereditarianism.[49] Against this we have to balance the concerted effort made by social hygiene groups to reach medical men in institutional positions, including the frequent addresses they gave to the annual conferences of MOHs.

Much depended on the composition of local government. More work needs to be done on this but undoubtedly London, Leicester and Birmingham were eugenic strongholds at one time. In Birmingham, Mrs Ellen F. Pinsent, member of the Royal Commission of 1908 and the Birmingham Heredity Society, was elected to the Birmingham Council in 1919. A.D. Steel-Maitland, a Birmingham MP and supporter of the 1913 Act was also a member of the Heredity Society. So were an influential local family, the Cadburys. Neville Chamberlain, later to become a Birmingham MP, Minister of Health and Prime Minister, was also a member. At that time, 1911, he was on the City Council and the management committee of the General Hospital.[50] The consequences of this can be seen in the appointment of W.A. Potts, a eugenicist, as official psychologist to the Birmingham Courts to assess those brought before them for mental deficiency — an experiment which it was hoped would be widely repeated. In other words, where the protagonists of social hygiene could establish a hold, they generated the experts they needed.

The other area where social hygiene and science overlapped was the top of the profession. Social hygienists included a great many doctors to the Royal Family — Sir Thomas Barlow, Sir Rickman Godlee, Sir Alfred Fripp and Lord Dawson of Penn. Dawson was created a baron in 1920 and a Viscount in 1936. He had been physician to a succession of Kings and had been chosen by the first Minister of Health, Christopher Addison, to be a government consultant. Dawson was a member of the CAMW, the birth control movement, and sympathetic to eugenics. He was also deeply involved in medical politics.[51]

Similarly Lord Horder, president for many years of the Eugenics Society, was a Royal physician. He counted two Prime Ministers, Bonar Law and Ramsay MacDonald, among his patients and in 1933 was created a baron. His interests are the complete exemplification of social hygiene. They included eugenics, smoke and noise abatement, the Boy Scouts, the General Council for Physical Recreation and the provision of National Parks. Along with physical fitness, purity of air and the preservation of the country went an interest in mental hygiene. He was a patron of the Child Guidance Clinic set up in 1927, and of the Society for the Study and Treatment of Delinquency. He was a family planner and member of the Institute of Management, Horder also founded in 1948 the Fellowship for Freedom in Medicine, set up to oppose the National Health Service.[52]

If social hygiene was not simply a means to advance the interests of scientists, did it have that function for women? Many of the organisations of social hygiene owed their existence to the dynamism and charisma of individual women — Dendy, Nethersole, Neville Rolfe and Evelyn Fox. The latter steered the CAMW throughout most of the years of its existence. None of these ladies had a professional training. They owed their positions to their abilities and interest in social questions.

The high representation of women reflects the origins of social hygiene in private charitable work. As these groups acquired 'expert' medical or scientific personnel the representation of women fell. In 1927, the lay committee of the People's League had 13 women out of 29 members. Their medical and scientific committees had 9 out of 96. The CAMW's executive in 1927 had 25 women members out of 70. Among its local organisations which relied on unpaid, voluntary work, 10 out of 16 representatives were women. The Eugenics Society had a high female membership of just over 40 per cent in 1937. Of these, only a small proportion were medically qualified although the proportion of the medically qualified in the Society as a whole was high. The National Council for Mental Hygiene, almost exclusively an organisation of medically qualified people, had no lay members and no women on its foundation.

There was a similar dearth in the NIIP largely because of its industrial bias. However Beatrice Edgell, Professor of Psychology at the University of London, was a member and so was Winifred Cullis who held the Sophia Jex-Blake Chair of Physiology of London University. In 1930, to redress this lack, the NIIP decided to found a women's section with Ruth Balfour and the Countess of Chichester. But although this contained a few independent professional women like the eugenicist and Fabian, Stella Churchill, and Winifred Cullis it was otherwise composed of the wives of existing members.[53]

However whilst the development of the social hygiene movement into broader organisations drawing on medical 'experts' reduced the influence of women in them, it also, paradoxically, increased the opportunities for paid professional work outside the home. These organisations both provided full-time paid posts and offered courses for the professional training of social workers. Frequently the chief beneficiaries were women. In this respect the social hygiene movement encouraged the entry of women into active professional life.

In addition social hygiene touched on questions of family life and sexual conduct. Some women argued for a more feminist perspective in these areas. Mrs Neville Rolfe and Elizabeth Sloan Chesser both appealed for the better treatment of the unwed mother. Elizabeth Sloan Chesser, in particular, wanted state assistance for the unsupported mother as well as regulation of the hours and conditions of women's work.[54] Both Mrs Neville Rolfe of the Social Hygiene Council (previously the National Council for Combatting VD) and Elizabeth Sloan Chesser attacked the double standard in sexual morality. They believed that a great wrong was done to the wife infected with VD by the husband and that this state of affairs should be put right by insisting on the same standard of sexual morality for men as for women. This was one, though not the only, reason why, under Rolfe's influence, the NCCVD was against treating VD by simply providing the medical means for avoiding it. This led to a breakaway from the NCCVD and the formation of the National Association for the Prevention of VD, which insisted in treating the question purely as one of prophylaxis and propaganda.[55]

The solution Chesser and Rolfe offered to the problem of the double standard was highly conventional. Neville Rolfe wanted her Council to strengthen family ties. Elizabeth Sloan Chesser wanted to enforce a single standard of morality on both sexes. She was against free love and easier divorce. Her ideal was romantic love followed by a lifetime of monogamy.[56] But then this was also the ideal professed by society at large.

These women in the social hygiene movement, drawn as they were from largely conventional middle class and upper class backgrounds, were usually socially conservative in their views. Even the interest of some in feminism was not universally shared. Among the ladies who petitioned for the Mental Deficiency Bill of 1913, were Mrs Arnold Toynbee, Louise Creighton, wife of the Bishop of London, Mrs T.H. Green and Lady Frederick Cavendish. These also signed the petition in the periodical *Nineteenth Century* against the extension of the suffrage to women.[57] Above all, even the female social hygienists who were feminists were often ferocious economic moralists of the old *laissez-faire* school. They were intent on making the working class family a self sufficient, economically independent unit with all the virtues of thrift and hard work said to be characteristic of the successful middle class.

If this was the case why did many on the left, particularly in the Labour movement, support social hygiene? In the parliamentary debates on the Mental Deficiency Bill, Leslie Scott described a deputation he had received from the Manchester and Salford Districts Trades and Labour Council petitioning in favour of the bill. Five Members of Parliament elected as representatives of the labour movement, responded to the call of the Eugenics Society and the COS in 1911 to help steer a mental deficiency bill through parliament. The five who attended the meeting called in the House of Commons for this purpose were George N. Barnes, Arthur Henderson, Joseph Pointer, Fred Jowett and William Crooks. Among those who, in addition to these, voted or supported the 1913 Mental Deficiency Bill were the Labour MPs Ramsay MacDonald, Charles W. Bowerman, James Parker, George H. Roberts, John E. Sutton, Frank Goldstone, W.T. Wilson, William Adamson and George Wardle.[58]

After 1918, support from within the Labour Party declined. But there was still a minority who, in 1931, voted for the sterilisation of mental deficients. In addition, Ernest Thurtle, a Labour MP between the wars, was a consistent advocate of birth control and served on the Workers Committee for Sterilisation set up by the Eugenics Society in the 1930s to win friends in the labour movement.[59] The 1931 Sterilisation Bill was introduced into the Commons by A.G. Church, Labour MP for Leyton East in 1923-24, and for Central Wandsworth in 1929-31. It was supported by R.D. Denman, Labour MP for Central Leeds (1929-31), and W.H. Dickinson also a Labour MP, who, when a Liberal in 1912, had introduced the Mental Defect Bill. If, as the saying has it, Labour is a loose coalition of interests what interests were represented by these

social hygienists? Close examination of these Labour members reveals
a number of interesting points about them. First, a high proportion of them
were on the right of the Labour Party. Second, they contain a higher than
average number of people who later broke away from the Labour Party.

After Joseph Pointer's election in 1908 the socialists in his constituency 'were constantly criticising his rapid shift to a moderate Labour
position'.[60] In particular he became very unpopular by supporting the
sentencing to gaol in 1912 of Thomas Mann for his anti-militarist pamphlet 'Don't Shoot!'. James Parker, Labour MP for Halifax (1906-18)
was one of the minority within the ILP who took a pro-war line on the
outbreak of war in 1914 and joined the Recruiting Committee set up by
the government. After the Labour movement — torn by dissension over
the war — broke with the war-time coalition in 1918, Parker remained
a minor official in the coalition government and stood at subsequent elections as Coalition Labour, a pseudonym for the patriotic pro-war
breakaways from the Labour Party. Similarly, George N. Barnes, already
in trouble with his union, the Amalgamated Society of Engineers, for
his support of the Liberal government's Labour Dispute bill, eventually
broke with the Labour Party over the war. He resigned in 1918 and in
the early 1920s became associated with the National Democratic Party
— a patriotic party for the working man.[61]

George H. Roberts took a similar path but his ultimate destination
in the 1920s was the Conservative Party for whom he eventually stood,
unsuccessfully, as a parliamentary candidate. Roberts was interested in
the birth control movement and appeared in 1923 as a witness for Marie
Stopes in her libel action against Dr Halliday Sutherland. He had read
'Benjamin Kidd, the most popular expositor of social Darwinism in the
early twentieth century'. The reasons he gave for support for birth control were that,

> It is a deplorable fact today that while the better-to-be possess this know-
> ledge and are, in my opinion, ordering their lives so as to give their
> children greater and fairer opportunities, the class to which I belong,
> grovelling in their ignorance, are still producing in excessive numbers
> a race which is not fitted for the Empire which we have to govern.[62]

John Edward Sutton, MP for East Manchester (1910-18) and Clayton,
Manchester (1922) was under fire from his constituency party before
1914 for being too pro-Liberal. When the war came he also supported
it and the Recruiting Committee subsequently set up. But Sutton remained
within the Labour movement as did Arthur Henderson and William

Crooks. Crooks, a Londoner, was a radical Liberal rather than a socialist. Crooks supported the Criminal Law Amendment (White Slave) Act and the amendment in favour of flogging. He also was pro-war and on its outbreak he led the Commons in the singing of the National Anthem. Henderson, like Goldstone and Bowerman, was also a supporter of the war and on the right of the Labour Party. Goldstone, a representative of the National Union of Teachers, was close to the problems of mental deficiency in the schools. But none of these left the Labour movement. Neither Fred Jowett, W.T. Wilson, nor William Adamson falls into this pattern.[63] But then William Adamson was famed for his taciturnity and made few public pronouncements. According to his Times Obituary 'silence was his strongest asset'.[64]

The war of 1914-18 gave sharper definition to the coalition of interests forming the Labour movement, pushing some to the right and others to the left. So did the crisis in 1931 when the Labour Prime Minister Ramsay MacDonald left the Labour Party to go into coalition with the Conservatives and Liberals. Out of the 1931 crisis came the National Labour Party representing MacDonald's supporters. A.G. Church, R.D. Denman and W.H. Dickinson followed him. W.H. Dickinson, in fact, had joined Labour in 1930 and left it for National Labour in 1931. When the Eugenics Society tried to use Church to influence the Labour Party in Parliament in 1931, they were warned 'to keep Church's name out of it in any dealings with the Labour Party' since his apostasy had made him very unpopular.[65]

What characterised the ideology of the Labour social hygienist was the appeal of the national ideal. As George Barnes put it in an apologia for the National Democratic Party, one which could also serve as such for the National Labour Party, 'Political enfranchisement and organisation has changed the whole situation. Labour is no longer outcast. Indeed it has won its way to citizenship, . . . the thinkers of all classes are agreed that the highest possible standard of living for the mass of the people is the ideal to be aimed at . . .'.[66] W.A. Appleton, member of the People's League and founder of a trade union movement which had broken away from the mainstream of trade unionism in protest against its 'unpatriotic' and 'class war attitudes', was 'an advocate of co-partnership as a means of reconciling the doings of wage earners and employers and of conferring to labour a status more worthy than that of a hired man'.[67]

The social hygienist in the Labour movement tended to be patriotic, less committed to an independent party of Labour, inclined to view militancy with suspicion except in defence of the nation, likely to see a future for a contented and prosperous working class within the existing system, given certain reforms, and attracted by the ideal of industrial cooperation. He or she might also see a clear distinction between the upright working man and the feckless, lazy and profligate dregs of industrial society. These social views clearly struck a chord among some of the working class for they were the staple of the anti-socialist papers directed at the working man like the *Empire Citizen*, for which Bishop D'Arcy wrote.

The trouble was, if the nation was now one, which one was it? The majority of the Labour movement had strong reservations about the possibility of the different social classes uniting in harmony. During the debate on the Mental Deficiency Bill in 1913, the constituents of George Wardle were reported to be 'thoroughly dissatisfied with his action over the Insurance Act, Labour Exchanges, Bill for the Feebleminded and his support for the Government's action in using the military during strikes'.[68] *Justice*, organ of the Social Democratic Federation, commented on this debate,

> Almost the only fighters left in the House are the individualist Radicals, Wedgwood, Martin and Co., who have fought an excellent rearguard action against the Mental Deficiency Bill. After the incident the other day where a pedlar was deemed mentally deficient by the magistrates, because he held socialist views, it behoved some of the Labour members at least to back Wedgwood.[69]

In fact, suspicion of social hygiene among the Labour movement grew as its character and tactics became clearer. This was particularly so once the Ministry of Health was established in 1919 and health statistics became part of the parliamentary battle. In 1913, the *Labour Leader*, newspaper of the ILP, quoted the Chief Medical Officer of Health, Arthur Newsholme, on the different rates of infant mortality between classes. It claimed, 'Dr Newsholme, himself, points out that overcrowded insanitary dwellings and low wages are the chief factors in the appalling loss of child life'.[70] In the 1920s, the Labour MP George Lansbury took up the same theme arguing in the health debates that the best health policy was an attack on poverty.

By 1929, however, when the debate on sterilisation was in full swing, it was clear to Lansbury that there was more than one attitude to the health statistics. There existed a lobby inside and outside Parliament which saw control of the fertility of the unfit as the means to eradicate poverty and ill-health. Lansbury was surprised and appalled at the tone of their remarks.

I want to say a word about the mentally deficient. It amuses me very much to read the newspaper articles and to listen to the experts in this House on the question of the mentally deficient.

I want to know where you will start to sterilise. I have never heard such utter rubbish and nonsense talked and written as I have heard and seen on this particular subject of the mentally deficient. I say before you are going to pick out — you doctors — those whom you will sterilise, take good care that we do not sterilise the lot of you first.[71]

There remained in Parliament, none the less, a small section of the Labour Party who actively advocated birth control and sterilisation. They tried to put the case for these measures without committing themselves to any of the social assumptions which had become attached to them. Ernest Thurtle, proponent of birth control, put the dilemma for Labour perfectly in a debate on the spread of birth control information.

I am a Socialist and I would be the last man to pretend that this restriction of families is any real cure for the root problem of poverty. The social inequalities and disabilities which afflict the mass of poor people have their roots much deeper than this. But even as a Socialist, I do say that knowledge which could enable working-class people to exercise a wise restriction in the size of their families would have an ameliorative effect on the condition of these workers, and it is for that reason that, as a Socialist, I am prepared to advocate this Bill.[72]

This was just the point. Social hygiene was offering a programme not just of health advice but an alternative to other forms of social amelioration. Could one take the information and leave behind the ideology? As the 1920s progressed and social hygiene developed, the issue became less and less easy to resolve.

Notes

1-3. Information about the following persons and families is taken from these sources: *Dictionary of National Biography*, 6 vols 1901-70 (Oxford University Press, Oxford, 1920-1981); *Who was Who?* 6 vols (Adam and Charles Black, London, 1920-1972); *Times Obituaries* 1951-75 (Newspaper Archive Developments Ltd, Reading, 1978); Joyce M. Bellamy and John Saville (eds), *Dictionary of Labour Biography*, 6 vols (Macmillan,

London 1972-1982). Their connection to social hygiene has been established from the following: Membership list of the CAMW (taken from the *Annual Report of the CAMW*, 1926-7); the Eugenics Society (from *Eugenics Review*, 1910-20 and *Annual Report* 1937-8; the National Council for Mental Hygiene (from the *BMJ*, 13 May 1922, pp. 771-2); the People's League of Health (Title page of Pamphlet, 1926 and *The Times*, 5 April 1937); the NIIP (from A.J. Welch and C.S. Myers, *Ten Years of Industrial Psychology* (Sir Isaac Pitman and Sons, London, 1932) pp. 107-111); the Mond-Turner participants from R. Charles, *The Development of Industrial Relations, 1911-39* (Hutchinson, London, 1973). In addition, affiliation has also been established from the voting for the Mental Deficiency Bill, H of C Deb, 29 July 1913, vol. 56, pp. 498-500; the letters to *The Times* in its support, 20 June 1912; 28 November 1912; 29 November 1912; 10 June 1913; 12 June 1913; Report of the Deputation to the House of Commons from the Eugenics Society and the National Association for the Feebleminded 15 July 1910 (Reported in *BMJ*, 16 July 1910, p. 147). Those asking Parliamentary questions in support of moving the Mental Deficiency Bills, 1910-13: Report of the meeting of the Eugenics Society and the National Association for the Feebleminded at the House of Commons, 5 December 1911, *Eugenics Review*, vol. 3 (1911-12). In addition, later involvement has been ascertained through the petition of the Grand National Council of Citizens in favour of sterilisation to the Ministry of Health, 16 February 1929 (MH58/103) and letters on the same to *The Times*, 3 February 1927, *Daily Mail*, 21 February 1929.

4. *Who was Who? 1929-40*, vol. 3, p. 1187.

5. Reginald Brabazon, 12th Earl of Meath, 1841-1929, *DNB 1922-30* pp. 100-1.

6. Rupert Guinness, Earl of Iveagh, ibid., *1961-70*, pp. 463-6.

7. Martin Wiener, *English Culture and the Decline of the Industrial Spirit, 1850-1980* (Cambridge University Press, Cambridge, 1980).

8. Leslie Scott, *Who was Who? 1941-50*, vol. 4, p. 1033 and *DNB 1941-50*, pp. 763-4.

9. Charles Bathurst, 1st Viscount Bledisloe, 1867-1958, *DNB 1951-60*, pp. 73-5.

10. Lady Aberdeen and Temair, 1857-1939, ibid., *1931-40*, pp. 348-9. Lady Aberdeen also founded the Women's National Association in 1907.

11. Sir Harry Lawson, 1st Viscount Burnham, 1862-1933, *DNB 1931-40*, pp. 533-4.

12. See *The Worker*, November 1910. This Conservative paper aimed at the working man was an offshoot of the Tariff Reform Workers Defence Union. It offered the working man smallholdings, better education, easier travel between city and suburbs, emigration and stopping immigration. For similarities with the programme of the eugenicists, see Editorial Notes, *Eugenics Review*, vol. 2 (1910)

13. R.A. Fisher, *The Genetical Theory of Natural Selection* (Clarendon Press, Oxford, 1930) pp. 250-61.

14. See W.C.D. Whetham, *Politics and the Land* (Cambridge University Press, Cambridge, 1927).

15. See W.E. Tanner, *Sir William Arbuthnot Lane* (Ballière, Tindall and Co., London, 1946).

16. Eug/D218, Eugenics Society Papers. File on Sterilisation.

17. Bristow, *Prostitution and Prejudice. The Jewish Fight against White Slavery, 1870-1939* (Schocken, New York, 1983).

18. William Boothby Selbie, 1862-1944, *DNB 1941-50*, pp. 768-9. John Scott Lidget 1834-53, ibid., *1951-60* pp. 633-5. He was an alderman of the LCC 1905-10, on their education committee, and leader of the Progressives on the LCC 1918-28.

19. Ellen F. Pinsent, 'Social Responsibility and Heredity' (read at the Church Congress, Cambridge, 1910). *National Review*, vol. 56 (1910) p. 507.

20. Eugenics and the Church, Editorial Notes, *Eugenics Review*, vol. 2 (1910), p. 162. See also report of the York Convocation, *The Times*, 29 November 1912.

21. See Notes 1-3; letter to *Daily Mail*, 1929; and Petition, 1929.

22. Eug/C10, C.P. Blacker to Baker, 15 February 1933.

23. Hensley Henson, *DNB 1941-50* pp. 378-9.

24. William Ralph Inge, 1866-1930, ibid., *1951-60*, pp. 529-32. Also, the Rt Rev. Lord William Gascoyne Cecil, Bishop of Exeter, *Who was Who? 1929-40*, vol. 3, p. 233.

25. Rt Rev. Ernest William Barnes, ibid., *1951-60*, vol. 5, p. 65.

26. Frederick D'Arcy, *Christian Ethics and Modern Thought* (Longman, Green and Co., London, 1912), p. 66.

27. See *The Empire Citizen*, 1921-22.

28. Barnes, 7 March 1937 in the *Northern Mail* and the *Newcastle Chronicle*. Reported in MH51/559 (Press cuttings).

29. M.J. Nolan, 'The Possibility of Limitation of Lunacy Legislation', *Journal of Mental Science*, vol. 52 (October 1906), pp. 756-65.

30. *Eyewitness*, 1 August 1912, pp. 193-4.

31. MH58/100-17 May 1935; MH58/101 14 March 1934; MH58/103 1929.

32. Mond, *DNB 1922-30*, pp. 602-5.

33. Quoted in Arthur Lucas, *Industrial Reconstruction and the Control of Competition* (Longman, Green and Co., London, 1937), p. 182.

34. See Chapter 6.

35. See *Eugenics Review*, vol. 3, 1912-13.

36. See Grand National Council of Citizens' Petition, MH58/103.

37. A. Mond, *Industry and Politics* (Macmillan, London, 1927), p. 70.

38. 'A National Plan for Britain', *Weekend Review*, 14 February 1931, p. iii.

39. See membership lists, Notes 1-3.

40. Howard Hazell was also prominent in the industrial profit sharing movement. See *Quarterly Review*, 1926.

41. See Eugenics Society Minute Books, 1930. Other bequests came from Leonard Darwin and Henry Twitchen. There were also anonymous donors.

42. G.E. Shuttleworth, *Mentally Deficient Children* (H.K. Lewis, London, 1895), pp. 110-11.

43. 'The Future of the Feebleminded', *BMJ*, 5 November 1898, p. 144.

44. 'The Case of the Feebleminded', ibid., 4 June 1892, p. 1214 (Committee appointed by the COS in 1890).

45. These included the provisions that the Act of 1899 should cease to be permissive, that the morally defective should be certifiable for one year and then annually, that after care committees should be formed, that all feebleminded incapable of self support or at large without proper control or means of subsistence or proved guilty of an offence should be placed under permanent care.

46. See William Chance, *The Better Administration of the Poor Law* (Sonnenschein and Co., London, 1895); *Old Age Pensions, The Better Way* (British Constitutional Association Pamphlet no. 10, London, 1907) Chance was a member of the London COS.

47. 'Legislation for the Feebleminded', *BMJ*, 16 July 1910, pp. 146-7.

48. See Arthur Newsholme, *Fifty Years in Public Health* (George Allen and Unwin, London, 1935) pp. 400-9.

49. For eugenic influence see M. Greenwood and J.W. Brown, 'An Examination of Some Factors Influencing the Rate of Infant Mortality', *Journal of Hygiene*, vol. 12 (1912), pp. 5-45.

50. See membership list of Birmingham Heredity Society in Eugenics Education Society, Fifth Annual Report, (1912-13), pp. 60-7.

51. Lord Dawson, 1864-1945, *DNB 1941-50*, pp. 201-4.

52. Lord Horder, 1871-1955, *DNB 1951-60*, pp. 501-3.

53. See Welch and Myers, *Ten Years of Industrial Psychology*, p. 114.

54. See Elizabeth Sloan Chesser, *Women, Marriage and Motherhood* (Funk and Wagnalls, New York and London, 1913).

55. See J. Austoker, *Biological Education and Social Reform. The BHSG 1925-42*, unpublished MA thesis, University of London, 1981. All of the council of the breakaway group, initially at least, were male.

56. Chesser, *Women, Marriage and Motherhood*.

57. *The Nineteenth Century*, vol. 25 (1889) p. 781.

58. See the House of Commons Meeting, 5 December 1911 (Reported in the *Eugenics Review*, vol. 3 (1911-12)), p. 355.

59. For the Workers Committee for Sterilisation, see Chapter 4. For Thurtle see his obituary, *The Times*, 23 August 1954, and his autobiography, *Time's Winged Chariot* (Chaterson, London, 1945). Thurtle was also connected with the Rationalist Press. His social origins were lower middle class. He was the son of a professional artist and a salesman and accountant in his youth.

60. Joseph Pointer, *DLB*, vol. 2, p. 302.

61. For Barnes, see ibid., vol. 4, pp. 7-15 and his autobiography, *From Workshop to War Cabinet* (Herbert Jenkins, London, 1923).

62. G.H. Roberts, *DLB*, vol. 4, p. 150.

63. For Sutton, Henderson, Goldstone, Crooks, *et al.*, see ibid., vols. 1-4. For Crooks's parliamentary interventions on white slavery see H of C Deb, 1 November 1912, vol. 43, p. 779.

64. *The Times* obit., 23 February 1936.

65. Eug/D215, Michael Pease to Blacker, September 1931. For A.G. Church see *Who was Who? 1951-60*, p. 210. For Denman see *Political Sketches* (Charles Thurman and Sons, Carlisle, 1948), and *Who Was Who? 1951-60*, p. 297.

66. Barnes, *From Workshop to War Cabinet*, pp. 300-1.

67. *The Times*, obit., 21 November 1940, p. 7.

68. Wardle, *DLB*, vol. 2, p. 374.

69. *Justice*, 2 August 1913, p. 4.

70. *Labour Leader*, 31 July 1913, Editorial.

71. Lansbury, H of C Debate, 1 May 1939, vol. 227, p. 1609.

72. Thurtle, H of C Deb, 9 February 1926, vol. 191, p. 851.

4 THE RATIONAL GOOD

> The kind of work in which you are engaged demands a not very com-
> mon combination of science and philanthropy. They are, as it were,
> moving hand in hand on the path of a most necessary hygenic process.
> (H.E. Ryle, Dean of Westminster, address at the inaugural meeting
> of the CAMW. *Journal of Mental Science*, vol. 63 (July 1917),
> p. 446.)

The foregoing chapter encompasses much of what social hygienists
thought and said but what did they do? In particular what was the relationship between social hygiene and contemporary scientific development? Three areas are important here: the development of industrial
psychology, the problem of nutrition and the question of mental
deficiency.

According to Sir Landsborough Thomson, historian of the Medical
Research Council, emotion rather than reason had dominated debate about
industrial conditions in the nineteenth century.

> Even in the long parliamentary battles fought during the nineteenth
> century upon the specific question of the reduction in the daily hours
> of work, battles fought between the advocates of a *laissez-faire* policy
> followed in the supposed interests of production and national wealth,
> on the one hand, and those pressing the claims of human charity upon
> the other, no appeal was made by either side to the laws of physiology
> or the test experiment.[1]

Sir Landsborough concluded that this had changed in the twentieth century with the establishment of the Industrial Fatigue Board, set up by
the government in the First World War, and the Institute of Industrial
Psychology, a private foundation founded in 1919 with grants from the
firm of Harrison Crosfield and the Carnegie Trust. These events, he
claimed, inaugurated the scientific approach to the question of the hours
and conditions of labour. This scientific approach combined physiology
and psychology. It was now possible to estimate what a worker needed
to eat in order to work efficiently and how fatigue could be mitigated
by shortening hours. Fatigue could also be diminished and productivity
increased by rearranging the workshop layout, lighting and work
materials.

These discoveries helped productivity. Sir Landsborough cited the case of Mather and Platt, the Manchester engineering firm, who, in an experiment in 1893, reduced working hours from 54 to 48 per week. This led to an increase in production and, during the First World War, the experiment was repeated in government-run arsenals and shipyards. This increase in efficiency and productivity was the justification for industrial psychology. However the mutual benefits for employers and employees were also stressed. C.S. Myers who left the Cambridge Psychology Laboratory in 1922 to head the National Institute of Industrial Psychology insisted that industrial psychology should not be confused with Taylorism which, in his view, involved merely a speeding up of the work process at the expense of the employee and was unpopular among the British workforce. To illustrate the benefits to the employee of industrial psychology, he cited two experiments conducted by the Institute for private employers in the first two years of its existence. The Institute had increased the power in the miners' lamps in a Lancashire coalfield and raised production and wages whilst lessening fatigue. They had raised output and wages in a sweet factory by reorganisation of the work materials and the work bench.[2]

By stressing these benefits, the proponents of industrial psychology hoped to win the confidence of the trade union movement. They were reasonably successful among a section of trade unionists. Walter Citrine, eventually chairman of the Trades Union Congress, C.T. Cramp of the National Union of Railwaymen and Arthur Pugh of the Iron and Steel Trades Confederation were members of the Institute of Industrial Psychology. What linked them to the Institute was, however, not merely the practical benefits they saw for the employee but the ideology of corporatism. These trade unionists were prominent in the Mond-Turner talks which took place in 1927-8, after the General Strike of 1926, between the trade union movement and a group of employers led by Sir Alfred Mond. These talks were intended to inaugurate an era of industrial peace by creating a system of joint consultation between the two sides of industry, which would meet regularly to iron out differences. Several of the firms involved in these negotiations were also prominent in the National Institute of Industrial Psychology.[3]

The government sponsored Industrial Health Board worked with the National Institute of Industrial Psychology in rather uneasy cooperation for a time. But the government body was concerned with specific and limited problems of health and fatigue. Only once, in what Sir Landsborough regarded as an unhappy experiment, did it attempt to advise on general questions of productivity and labour relations. The

National Institute of Industrial Psychology had, however, much broader aims. L. Urwick, a member of the Institute and head of the School of Business Management of Geneva, argued that industrial psychology was just one aspect of scientific management. As ownership of industry became separated from its control and direction a new professionally trained management was required. This would have to be selected by appropriate psychological tests and trained in the principles of business organisation.[4] The problems of business administration became more acute as rationalisation created larger and less manageable conglomerations. This led to further problems. C.S. Myers, in particular, pointed out the remoteness of employer and employee brought about by the end of the old-fashioned entrepreneur who both owned and ran a business and was personally known to his workforce. Scientific management could tackle this problem and devise various means to overcome alienation between management and labour.[5]

C.S. Myers found social Darwinism useful to theorise these developments. Small businesses were single-cell organisations, cartels were polyps. Evolution created differentiation and interdependence in the business organism. Industrial psychology was one of the means to bind together the different parts of the business organism and to prevent it from becoming too unwieldy. Thus as industrial evolution progressed so would the need for scientific management.[6] Myers saw corporatism as the social ideology of modern industry. He argued that ultimately not only would industry operate through joint councils peacefully settling disputes but that wealth would be divided in this way, 'allocation being determined by a joint council, representative of all concerned in their formation, and acting in the capacity of co-partnership, in the industry'.[7] Myers also saw vocational testing as a means to legitimise stratification between management and worker in industry.

> Especially after the experiences of the war, for good or evil, class distinctions are breaking down and the former hard and fast line of cleavage and opposition between management and labour must disappear in the cause of social evolution. Leadership and management must continue to exist but respect must be transferred from mere social position to personal efficiency.[8]

The National Institute of Industrial Psychology was involved from its inception in the development of vocational selection. In 1921 its scientific committee included Dr William Brown, Wilde Reader in Mental Philosophy at Oxford; Cyril Burt, eventually to become Professor of

Psychology in the University of London; Charles Spearman, Grote Professor of Mind and Logic, London; G.H. Thomson, Professor of Education at Edinburgh University; James Drever, Professor of Psychology, University of Edinburgh; Percy Nunn, Professor of Education, University of London; C.W. Valentine, Professor of Education at Birmingham; T.H. Pear, Professor of Psychology, University of Manchester; Beatrice Edgell, Professor of Psychology, University of London and F.C. Bartlett, Professor of Experimental Psychology at Cambridge. With this formidable array of psychologists *in situ*, the National Institute inevitably gave considerable encouragement to the spread of mental testing.

The Institute spent much of its time in devising and offering courses for industrial personnel officers, teachers and career guidance officers[9] in how to conduct mental tests. Cyril Burt did a good deal of this work. Round about the same time he was also drawing conclusions about the relationship between IQ and occupation. By the 1920s a considerable amount of work had been done correlating the two. The Institute, however, wanted tests not merely to indicate level of intelligence but those of a specific vocational nature. In the 1920s one of the first experiments along these lines was Burt's test for civil service typists. By the end of the 1930s Myers recorded a number of basic research findings along these lines, for example, the correlation between scores in tests of space perception with prognosis of suitability for engineering occupations.[10]

In the committee on Rationalisation set up by the Government Economic Advisory Council in August 1931, the Institute gave evidence on the need for industrial psychology and vocational selection, particularly in the realms of higher management. The officials from the Board of Education who gave evidence to the committee, however, considered the predictive value of a conventional educational qualification satisfactory.[11] None the less, some government departments used the services of the Institute's vocational selection procedure. In addition the Institute relied on openings from sympathetic education officials in local government for their projects. Among local education officials in their membership were P.B. Ballard, Robert Blair, G.H. Gater, C.W. Kimmins and F.H. Spencer of the London County Council. Birmingham Education Committee started a scheme for assessing applications for apprenticeships under the direction of the NIIP in 1927.

To Myers, a world in which vocational selection existed was not only more efficient but happier. This is surprising in view of the fact that, in one major survey conducted by the Institute, 55 per cent of the vocationally selected had different career ambitions from those selected for them.[12] Ultimately, however, Myers argued, vocational selection reduced the friction and unhappiness which arose when an individual was placed in an unsuitable working environment. This, together with the incorporation of the worker into joint consultative machinery and profit sharing, would, Myers believed solve contemporary industrial unrest. If this seems an unduly sentimental and optimistic view of industrial development, it has to be put side by side with another aspect of industrial psychology. Lurking behind the happy well adjusted worker was the 'ragged army', the dissatisfied, disobedient, unemployable and often mentally deficient employee.

> The mentally unstable employee is an irritant to his fellows and a nuisance to management. His kind is responsible for much of the existing unemployment and labour turnover. Ever worthless, himself, he is continually being discharged from one job to another as a worthless worker. He becomes more and more unfitted for a normal environment and finally joins the ranks of the unemployable, the alcoholic, the criminal and the insane.
>
> We now know that by the timely application of psychotherapeutic measures and by judicious selection of the environment such workers can, like early tuberculosis, be prevented from going downhill.[13]

At this point the task of industrial psychology shades off into mental hygiene and mental deficiency policy. As we shall see, the participants in the National Institute of Industrial Psychology interested themselves in these questions.

Industrial psychology rapidly became part of the task of social hygiene. C.S. Myers was a regular participant in the lecture programme of the People's League of Health.[14] The early programme of the National Council for Mental Hygiene included a commitment to study the individual in the industrial environment and speakers from the National Institute of Industrial Psychology were included in the conferences they organised. In 1926, Sir Lynden Macassey, a member of the Institute, spoke on the role of industrial psychology to the New Health Society.[15] He argued that the loss in production from sickness in Britain amounted to one-fifth of its annual national income. The Health groups should, therefore, work in tandem with the Institute to bolster industrial productivity by reducing avoidable sickness whilst the Institute increased the efficiency of the worker on the job. The National Council for Mental Hygiene also took up this theme. They believed the introduction of vocational selection was an important step in reducing psychomatic and emotional disturbance at work.[16]

The People's League was deeply concerned with industrial problems. On several deputations to the Ministry of Health in the 1920s the League asked for certificates of physical fitness to be mandatory for children leaving school to join the labour force and they also suggested periodic examination of the adult work force.[17] The government successfully avoided these schemes on the grounds of the liberty of the individual and the more pressing question of cost. The People's League was also concerned with the much broader question of unemployment. They led three deputations to the government on this issue, in 1922, 1927 and 1928. The policy they advocated was not increase of unemployment benefits or poor relief. The view the League took was highly orthodox as far as the level of unemployment benefit was concerned. In 1922, Sir Bruce Bruce-Porter, a member of the League, argued,

> At the present moment we as a nation are very hard up, and any attempt to make a grant of money along the lines to correspond to the pay of these days would soon land us in a state of bankruptcy and the conditions of the people would then be much worse.[18]

None the less, the People's League accepted that a decline in health was brought about by a rise in unemployment. This included mental health. During the delegation, Dr W.A. Potts, the Birmingham Court psychologist, attributed 'certain psychological disorders which manifested themselves either in revolutionary agitation or in moral delinquency, to ill-health caused by insufficient food'.[19] The solution the League suggested was twofold. They argued for a more productive use of the dole to mitigate the demoralising effects it had. This involved public works of various kinds and a tantalising reference by a representative of the League, Captain Donald Simson of the British Legion, to the scheme devised by Alfred Mond, Lord Melchett, in the 1920s for a premium to employers who took on idle hands.[20] The second suggestion was that of Sir Bruce Bruce-Porter who advocated food tickets for the unemployed in lieu of money. This was to regulate the unemployed's eating habits for, argued Sir Bruce Bruce-Porter, they spent unwisely because they were ignorant of food values. This issue, food values, diet and health, was to absorb increasing amounts of attention in the 1920s.

It was an observable fact that one reason for working was to get money for food. It was also true that one ate in order to work. This statement had, by the outbreak of the First World War, received scientific sanction. By then it was established that food had calorific value, that is, it produced heat when burned and when burned by the body's metabolism it produced energy for activity. It became possible to compare the calorific values of foodstuffs — the amount of heat each produced — and it also became possible to relate the expenditure of energy to the consumption of energy-producing food. In addition, it was established that the repair of tissue and the healthy growth of the body depended upon the amount of protein in a diet. Protein and calorific value became two important guides for nutritional scientists in estimating the adequacy or inadequacy of a particular diet.[21]

During the First World War, work was done in Britain and the USA on the calorific value of diets among different classes of the community, and among workers engaged in various occupations. From this emerged the practice of fixing scales of calorific values for different kinds of work. In 1918 a Medical Research Council Report quoted a set of standards worked out by the United States Department of Agriculture.[22] According to this a sedentary worker needed 2,700 calories per day, one involved in light work 3,000, in moderate work 3,500 and in hard physical work 4,500. The Royal Society produced their own estimates. These ranged from a tailor needing 2,750 calories to a stonemason who needed 4,850.[23] A research worker who estimated the diets of Glasgow families before and during the First World War, found the following fluctuations. Before the war the average adult in a Glasgow family consumed 110 grams of protein and 3,163 calories per day. During the war this had changed to 102 grams of protein and 3,298 calories.[24]

The difficulties of arriving at a precise figure are illustrated by these different estimates. Partly this was due to the fact that they were arrived at by observing what an individual in his day to day life consumed — which changed according to social, cultural and economic circumstances. Second, any generalisation about the optimum figure included the researchers' own assumptions about behaviour and cultural expectations. But the figures provided roughly fell within a range sufficiently uniform to allow it to become a means to analyse the adequacy of diet.

In Britain, E.P. Cathcart, a physiologist at Glasgow University, member of the Industrial Fatigue Board and the National Institute of Industrial Psychology, was closely associated with the development of this aspect of nutritional science. The Cathcart scale became commonly referred to as a tool of nutritional analysis in Britain. Cathcart was also deeply involved in the social and political consequences of applying this nutritional scale. In 1922 and 1923, during a period of struggle in the coalfields over wages, Labour MPs raised the question of the adequacy of miners' wages in Parliament. There was, at this time, much talk of malnutrition in the coalfields. In direct response to this, Cathcart undertook a study for the Medical Research Council into the nutrition of miners and their families which appeared in 1924.[25] In it he used a comparison of the actual calorific value of the diet of the adult miner with the projected number of calories they would need to do their work efficiently.

Cathcart took 3,400 calories as the amount needed and he studied diet in five mining districts, Durham, Derby, Northumberland, Lancashire and Stirling. In four of these the standard of 3,400 calories was not reached. Cathcart, however, did not draw the conclusion that wages were inadequate. Instead, he argued that extraneous factors were responsible for the low calorific value of these miners' diets. He listed a history of interrupted work through strikes, husbands who cheated on housekeeping money and above all bad housekeeping as the chief contributory causes for the shortfall. Moreover, a few years later in 1926 Paton and Findlay went further and revised the scale of calorific value down. 'In this study the observable intake of calories per man per day was 2,600 in the Scottish districts studied.'[26] They concluded therefore that,

The usually accepted 3,000 calories by Lusk's standard as the minimum requirement per man per day for the family diets of our population, more than 80 per cent of whom are town dwellers, is excessive and that from 2,500-2,700 calories is nearer to the correct figure, ie, that the standard might be reduced by 10 or possibly 20 per cent.[27]

The political and social implications of fixing diets scientifically in an era of struggle over wages were obvious. But the whole issue of nutrition became more complicated after the discovery of 'accessory food factors' or vitamins. This had important implications for the study of the causes of rickets, a bone deforming disease attacking children. This condition was particularly a disease of the poor. There were in the first two decades of the twentieth century a number of practical, common-sense remedies advocated for its cure, of which the intake of cod liver oil was one. But no exact aetiology of rickets existed and certainly no accepted theory of causation. The concept of a 'deficiency' disease, that is a disease caused by deficiency of diet, was not easily accepted. But in the first years of the century research workers began to identify specific chemical elements in food whose absence from the diet was associated with disease.[28] Between 1918 and 1921, Edward Mellanby identified rickets as a deficiency of fat-soluble vitamin D which aided calcification and of vitamin A which helped growth.

Mellanby's work was by no means universally accepted. In the first place certain problems arose because initially vitamins A and D were not identified as separate nor their different functions identified. Therefore the opponents of the theory could point to diets apparently rich in fats that did not cure rickets. Second, the transformation of the precursors contained in the fat into the vitamin takes place in the body under the influence of sunlight. This brought into sharp focus the conflict which existed between two schools of thought on rickets, the sunlight and fresh air theory and the dietary deficiency one.

Much of what doctors thought about rickets before the identification of vitamin D was the result of encounters they had with families in whom the disease was prevalent. The trouble was that there were many social characteristics which could be enumerated in these families. One persistent characteristic was poverty, endemic or intermittent. But there were others. The leading proponents of the fresh air and sunshine theory were Noel Paton, Professor of Physiology at Glasgow University, 1906-28, and Leonard Findlay, Professor of Pediatrics, Glasgow University. Findlay believed in an infection theory of rickets brought about by overcrowding. Paton believed in similar causes.[29] In his opinion insanitary and squalid conditions caused rickets and it could be cured by cleanliness, fresh air and sunshine. They could point to evidence to support their views which correlated cubic air space per person and home conditions with rickets.[30]

Even before the impact of vitamin research, however, their views were not generally accepted. If overcrowding and rickets correlated, so too did poor diet and rickets and some researchers plumped for poorness of diet even before any scientific demonstration of its relationship to the disease. There was also another dimension to this argument. What caused rickets determined the kinds of social policies pursued. The implications of the work done by Harold Corry Mann for the MRC on rickets was that it was a disease of poverty and low wages.[31] In 1922 he published research done on the families of London dock labourers in 1919 and 1920. He firmly related the incidence of rickets to type of diet and the type of diet to the income per head of the family. He also argued that income was determined by social conditions such as family size, regul-arity of employment, level of wages and absence of the chief breadwinner. The picture of London dock labouring families he painted in his report was of a responsible group of mothers whose capacity to feed their families was dependent on the level of employment available and the rate of wages, not on what was to become a powerful counter-attack to his views, their efficiency or inefficiency. Corry Mann also praised the work of the mother-and-child welfare clinics which distributed cheap milk.

In contrast the work of Paton and Findlay argued against dietary deficiency and poverty as the causes of rickets. The social solutions they offered were rehousing, better hygiene among mothers in the care of the home and a regime of exercise and fresh air. They also denigrated the value of the free clinics in helping to improve the condition of rickety children.[32] Paton and Findlay served on the Scottish Child Life Investigation Committee which was part of the Child Life Investigation set up in 1919 by the MRC (of which Paton was a member, 1918-23) to look into the sociological aspects of child disease and mortality. They continued to exercise influence on this investigation throughout the 1920s.

In the light of the work of Mellanby and others on dietary deficiency we have to ask why they continued to exercise such influence? By 1926, for example, the *BMJ* whilst accepting Mellanby's researches still plumped for sunlight as the predominant factor in prevention of rickets.[33] This coincided with a craze for treatment by ultraviolet lamps. Others were even more sceptical of deficiency theory. Leonard Hill, a physiologist at the National Institute for Medical Research, member of the MRC and of the People's League, argued at the League's conference on Sunlight and Health in 1925, that 'rickets in children could be cured by it (sunlight) even if a bad diet was not changed'.[34] In 1930, in exasperation at the obduracy of some of his colleagues, Mellanby spoke out,

> With all the good will in the world, even if we were prepared to go about naked, we would find it difficult in England to procure from the sun enough ultra violet radiation to keep our bones straight and well calcified. It cannot be too much emphasized that rickets can be completely prevented . . . independently of sunlight, if sufficient vitamin D is included in the diet from birth and prenatally in the mother's diet.[35]

The attractions of sunlight as a health policy were several. First, the rare incidence of sunlight in Britain, particularly in the smoke-filled industrial areas, was seen as sufficient to account for the prevalence of the disease in the industrial population. It also explained its seasonal variation. There were, however, other more ideological reasons. The advocacy of sunlight and fresh air was strongly linked to the philosophy of the natural. C.W. Saleeby, the eugenicist, was also a founder of the Sunlight

League. He advocated the discarding of restricting clothes, the exposure of the body to sun and air and, in parentheses, the abandonment of prudery and self consciousness. He said very little about vitamins. Saleeby became a member of Arbuthnot Lane's New Health Society and he gave the ideas of that organisation good copy in the *New Statesman*, where he wrote a health column under the title 'Lens'.

This emphasis on sunlight and fresh air as a curative had other causes. It was part of the sense of 'place' which J. A. Thomson had talked about in his digressions on social hygiene. This sense of 'place' had grown along with Britain's industrial areas. It was born of fear of the city and the desire to recreate in Britain the social ties of the country. Arbuthnot Lane's New Health Society went to extreme lengths to bring this about by advocating resettlement on the land. Other groups contented themselves with schemes for the suburban resettlement of the working class, for allotments and gardens and for the provision of open spaces and parks. These views were mixed up with the hope that the countryside, or its urban facsimiles, might soothe the excited, debilitated, nervous urban proletariat. In addition, the denizens of the Empire hoped that fresh air and exercise might create the stuff out of which Empires were maintained.

These ideas rather than social reformism animated the sunlight and fresh air school. It is true that Paton's work suggested that slum clearance and rehousing were important preventatives of rickets. But rehousing was a major plank in Conservative party programmes offered to the working class before and after 1914 and largely non-controversial. Christopher Addison, the first Minister of Health (Alfred Mond was the second) served on the MRC with Paton and Findlay and he certainly believed a rehousing programme would be a major contribution to health. During his time as Minister of Health he became deeply involved in the question of housing.[36] But in Britain in the 1920s, it was wages and unemployment which were controversial. Would an improvement in wages lead to an improvement in health? Cathcart, Paton, Findlay and others engaged on the Scottish Child Life Investigation went to great lengths to prove that it would not.

The People's League of Health had strong proponents of sunlight and air on its medical council including Sir Bruce Bruce-Porter who considered that the majority of cases of physical unfitness were due to their lack. Leonard Hill and Robert McCarrison, two nutritionists who served on the People's League, were also convinced of their prime importance. The People's League cooperated with the Sunlight League in the late

1920s to get the government to pass a measure of smoke abatement (as well as noise control) on the grounds of the importance of sunlight to health. They were also, like the New Health Society, deeply involved in questions of the purity of food and control of additives. Eventually these issues led the People's League to throw itself in the 1930s into the campaign for purer tuberculin-tested milk. They campaigned to make the conditions of milk production and distribution more hygienic and to rid Britain's dairy herds of bovine tuberculosis.

These were extremely useful measures. However, there remained the thorny question of diet and its adequacy for those on low incomes. In 1925, the People's League set out to show 'How the Working Man's Family can be well fed at present wage rates'.[37] In their pamphlets on good feeding they set out a series of diets for the working class family. The average weekly working class income was estimated at £120 per annum (assuming 48 weeks out of 52 were worked). This gave 50s (£2 10s) per week for food, rent and other expenditures. Contemporary estimates of average annual earnings in 1925 have put the earnings of agricultural labourers at around £75 per annum, the average wage in manufacturing industry at £131 per annum and that in the mining industry at around £134 per annum.[38] These last two estimates are inflated because they lump together all employed grades whether skilled, administrative or unskilled. They also assume continuous employment for 48 weeks. None the less, taking these facts into consideration, the People's League estimate of an average working class wage was reasonably accurate.

The problem was, as the Medical Research Council Reports of the period show, a substantial number of working class family incomes fell below that figure. Cathcart and Murray's study of working class families in Cardiff and Reading in 1928 (published in 1932) showed that out of the 113 families studied, 20 had an income of between £1 and £1 19s 11d a week (a mean of £1 13s 7¼d). A further 50 families had an income of between £2 and £2 19s 11d (a mean of £2 7s 5d) in Reading and £2 10s 7¼d in Cardiff.[39] Thus, 70 families out of 113 were earning or receiving below or just around the average. In addition the People's League budget allowed for a father, mother and two children only. They also gave a rather low figure for rent, 7s per week. Cathcart and Murray gave the figures for rent as 13s 3d in Cardiff and 9s 9d in Reading. Corry Mann in 1919-21 estimated the average rent in London was 10s per week although admittedly rents were higher in the capital city.

The People's League estimated the total expenditure on food in a family of four receiving 50s (£2 10s) per week as 25s 6d (£1 5s 6d) or

8s 6d each for two adults and 8s 6d for two children. Although the menu they drew up left out a staple of working class consumption and social life — tea — and allowed for fresh meat on only three days in the week, it was reasonably varied. Perhaps in recognition of the fact that because of higher rent, a larger family, unemployment or a lower income, many working class families would fall below this figure, the People's League provided alternative diets at 7s 2d per adult, 6s 7d and even 5s 11d.

The labour-saving diet at 7s 2d dropped fresh meat, tea and vegetables (apart from a bunch of watercress). The staple was bread and margarine. Jam appeared mysteriously on the menu although it was not included in the cost. Corned beef, cheese and eggs were the sources of protein and fat, together with a small amount of butter. Nine oranges and six bananas added fruit and variety.

The potato diet at 6s 7d per head required a stout constitution. The family suppers consisted of mashed potatoes, bread, margarine and milk on Sunday, cold sliced potatoes on Monday, baked potatoes on Tuesday, bread, margarine and milk on Wednesday, potato and cheese pie on Thursday, potato soup with dumplings and bread on Friday and potato and cheese cakes on Saturday. The only meat was herrings, minced ox heart and corned beef. The fare of the family on 5s 11d per adult was even worse. They were advised to take the potato diet minus the onions, sugar, cabbage, tomatoes, cress and oranges which enlivened it. This diet had no fresh meat, no eggs, no fruit or vegetables, no tea or sugar, nor even a cheering sausage or piece of bacon.

These diets put aside all aesthetic or social considerations. They regarded the stomach as something to be bent to the exigencies of the wage system. At the lower levels they were not even healthy. The People's League, given the choice, were not inclined to adopt it themselves. Leonard Hill, for example, advised better off audiences that a healthy diet should consist of a breakfast of eggs, bread and butter, milk and jam, or porridge, milk and fruit; a dinner of meat, potatoes, greens and a pudding; a tea of meat, or eggs or cheese and milk pudding and fruit.[40] This he regarded as modest, yet it was unattainable on the People's League's most generous estimate of expenditure. A double standard of eating was, therefore, advocated. The middle classes sat down to first class protein daily in the form of meat, fish or eggs. The poor sat down, even on the best diet, to sheep's head broth at least once a week.

In addition, how necessary was this advice? The working class diet already adapted itself to the available resources. Corry Mann reported how, as their income for food fell, housewives replaced dripping, suet, lard, butter and bacon fat by margarine. When their income fell even further, they replaced margarine by treacle and the consumption of bread and potatoes rose. In good times, butter, fresh milk, (as opposed to tinned condensed milk), eggs, bacon and fresh meat reappeared. At rock bottom these same families survived on a diet of potatoes, bread, golden syrup, broth from scraps and a brew of tea (from repeated boilings of the leaves) sweetened with condensed milk.[41] Other expedients were 'tick' or credit to tide them over and, as Cathcart reported in Glasgow, the use of tobacco to depress the appetite.

In fact, the management of diet to fit income already went on. What the People's League diet sheets did was state a political not a scientific principle. They were a demonstration of the adequacy of the present wage system and they threw aside all considerations of pleasure, satisfaction and tradition in their determination to prove that survival was possible on current wages.

Would good domestic management improve the health of the working classes? This question was significant in medical sociology in the 1920s, and in society at large. The connection between social class and ill-health was already well known. Paton and Findlay in their reports for the Medical Research Council in 1926 on 'Poverty, Nutrition and Growth' listed five studies from 1833 to 1913 which set out the differing incidences of mortality and ill health in social classes.[42] In spite of improvements in public health these differences persisted. Were they due to poverty? Views differed but a strong body of opinion regarded domestic management as the most important factor. The term 'maternal inefficiency' which was coined before the First World War continued to be widely used in medical literature in the 1920s and, to some extent, in the 1930s too. In addition, this term 'maternal inefficiency', which suggested that teaching and propaganda was an important weapon for improving health, began to acquire, in some hands, an increasingly pessimistic, hereditarian interpretation. In other words, it was suggested by some researchers that maternal inefficiency was often caused by low intelligence and therefore it was a largely intractable problem. At least, education alone could not solve it.

These concepts found their way into the medical research literature of the 1920s and early 1930s. After the First World War, in 1919, the Medical Research Council instituted, among other things, a project on the study of nutrition and one on child life. The child life study was divided into two. In Scotland, Paton and Findlay looked at sociological aspects. In England, the research was orientated towards the pathology of childhood disease. Paton and Findlay published the results of their study in 1926, *Nutrition, Poverty and Growth*. In this work, the reasons for differential mortality and growth patterns between social classes were examined, and the question of nutritional influences brought up. Paton and Findlay rejected the idea that racial influences could account for the differences in stature and physique between social classes. This theory had lingering influence in the 1920s. Paton and Findlay did not altogether reject it. They hypothesised that natural selection might have produced a 'small, machine-tending' workman and a wife, also small who 'did not need much food'.[43] But they accepted the influence of environmental factors such as nutrition on the height and weight of working class children. What they did not accept was the attribution of this to poverty and low incomes. Instead they argued that what distinguished the homes with poverty and bad conditions was the 'inefficiency' of the mother, and they considered this inefficiency to stem from poor mental endowment.

> What is not demonstrated is that simple increase of income would be followed by improvement in the condition of the children. Bad parents irrespective of their income tend to select bad houses as the money is often spent on other things. The saying that 'What is the matter with the poor is poverty' is not substantiated by these investigations (which) indecisive as many of them are, indicate that a position must be taken up removed from that of the sociological or political theorist who believes that a simple increase of income would remedy all evils and from that of a thorough going eugenist on the other. The evidence supports neither extreme but seems to indicate that current teaching gives too much rather than too little weight to environmental factors which, theoretically at least, it might be possible to remedy by economic adjustments.[44]

Paton and Findlay's theory of maternal inefficiency was taken up by Cathcart and Murray in the two studies on nutrition they did for the MRC in 1931 and 1932.[45] They altered the concept slightly. In 1926, they argued, too much weight had been given to maternal as opposed to paternal inefficiency. Inefficiency was just as much a product of bad fathers as it was of bad mothers. But the hereditarianism had hardened. The parentally inefficient were definitely recruited from the unfit. 'We believe it is essential to recognise that a physical segregation has taken place. The weaker and less effective members of society do and must gravitate to the bottom of the economic scale'.[46] It was a case of the chicken and the egg. Although Cathcart and Murray discovered that poverty was an index of ill-health, was poverty the cause of that ill-health? Whilst conceding this to be so in some cases, the brunt of their argument was that mental inefficiency leading to bad domestic management was a major contributory factor. That is why some families, in their opinion, rose above poverty by thrift and good housekeeping whilst others succumbed.

Shepherd Dawson, a psychologist with close connections with eugenics, produced an MRC report on 'Intelligence and Disease' which tried to prove this by experiment. Dawson, in his investigation with J.C.M. Coon in 1931 found, 'The outcome of the inquiry was very remarkable, for as regards these children it was found that of the various external factors which were studied maternal efficiency . . . was the only one which played a significant part in determining nutrition in the child.'[47] Dawson's work was something of a departure for he attempted to find a direct correlation between IQ and ill-health with the hope of further elucidating the supposed connection between mental inefficiency and physical inefficiency. This proved, in this particular study, to be a very weak connection however.

The pervasiveness of the idea of parental inefficiency is explained by the significance given to eugenics in the 1920s and, in particular, the eugenic explanation of social problems. In 1910, E.J. Lidbetter, under the direction of the Eugenics Society, began to assemble his pedigree of pauper families to prove that poverty was the product of poor mental endowment, and an hereditary condition. The Eugenics Society promulgated the idea that a rigorous policy of institutionalisation of the 'feebleminded' would lead to a diminution of various social problems including pauperism. In their hands mental deficiency policy became not merely a solution for individual problems but a means of social engineering, involving the cure of many social evils.

Their view was widely accepted. The New Health Society believed that the key to social progress was heredity and nutrition. They had friendly relations with the Eugenics Society. Writing in 1928, an official of the Eugenics Society remarked 'Hitherto we have worked very cordially together, they have given us some space for Eugenics articles in their Journal and there has been talk of our lecturing for them in some courses they arrange.'[48] Sir Arthur Keith was, in fact, the New Health Society's expert on eugenics and his pessimistic views on the decline of civilisations due to uncontrolled heredity must have chimed in well with aspects of their anti-modernism.

The People's League was also sympathetic to eugenics. From its foundation Olga Nethersole was concerned about the propagation of the 'unfit'.[49] In 1925 they held a series of lectures on Mental Health. Sir Frederick Willis, a member of the People's League, CAMW and National

Council for Mental Hygiene argued, 'one of the most important things they could do was to try and stop the growth of the mentally deficient population. . . . In the end, it was going to imperil our national welfare, unless it was dealt with.'[50] The People's League's experts on eugenics and mental deficiency were A.F. Tredgold and W.A. Potts, both members of the Eugenics Society. Potts, one of the Eugenics Society's earliest members and lecturers, was official psychologist to the Birmingham courts. In that role he examined for mental deficiency and mental disorder every suspect who came before them. It was due to Potts's influence that the People's League became committed to the extension of the 'Birmingham System' in all criminal cases. They were particularly interested in the use of psychologists in children's courts. In the mid-1920s, the People's League pressed the government for an amendment to the Children's Act of 1908 to get the condition of encephalitis lethargica recognised in children brought before the courts as a physical illness which affected mental condition. They were also keen on the extension of psychological testing and examination to the school as well as the court. This psychological examination included specifically the identification and treatment of the 'feebleminded'.[51]

Their interests in this sphere in the 1920s corresponded to those of the National Council for Mental Hygiene. This group was largely formed of prominent members of the Royal Medico-Psychological Association which included both psychiatrists and psychologists within its ranks. Most British psychologists at that time had medical degrees as well as training in psychology. The precepts of the National Council were to encourage the development of the mental sciences and to strive for their adoption in medical schools and elsewhere.[52] Like the People's League they were concerned with 'normal' mental development as well as the insane and mentally deficient. Sir Maurice Craig, their first president, insisted that the future for the mental sciences lay in counselling the family, the school and later the adult and the provision of better mental health facilities (including industrial psychology). At the same time its research programme in 1921 included the study of the relationship between heredity and environment although a great deal of their time was taken up with theories of the pitfalls of ordinary emotional development (W.A. Potts specialised in a kind of potted Freudianism in talking about the emotional abnormality of criminals). In this way, they added something new to the discourse of health in the 1920s.

The National Council for Mental Hygiene was, none the less, concerned with mental deficiency. Its first committees included one on Mental Deficiency in which Potts and Tredgold played an important role.

Evelyn Fox, secretary of the CAMW, also featured prominently in the mental hygiene movement. Other prominent eugenicist members of the National Council's Committee included Sir Humphrey Rolleston, Bryan Donkin, Nathan Raw, Doris Odlum, Bernard Hart, C.S. Sherrington and C.S. Myers.[53] Most of those involved in the mental hygiene movement had also been important in the campaign for the 1913 Mental Deficiency Act. The National Council for Mental Hygiene was one of the first to come out in favour of the Eugenics Society's campaign in favour of sterilisation.

This campaign was brought about by what the social hygienists conceived of as the failure of the 1913 Act to reduce or eradicate mental deficiency. Because of lack of funds and the dilatoriness of some local authorities, provision for institutionalisation was considered to have fallen behind needs. There was considered to be a good proportion of people who needed, but had escaped, certification. In addition many of those certified as mental deficients were outside institutions on licence — that is allowed out under restricted conditions, in particular, under guardianship. Since its inception in 1913 (with a pause during the war) the CAMW had served as an agency for referring possibly certifiable people to institutions and providing guardians under the licence system. They also received a grant from the Exchequer (£2000 in March 1921) for their work in training social workers and general practitioners in the principles of mental deficiency policy. Each year their journal recorded the number of certifications for which they were responsible.[54]

The general feeling in the CAMW was that the problem was only being touched on. In 1927, together with the Eugenics Society and the Board of Control, they got an amendment passed in Parliament — again opposed by Wedgwood — to make certification easier by removing the obligation on the part of the certifying medical man or woman to prove defect from birth or a very early age. They also joined the People's League in the campaign over encephalitis lethargica. But the CAMW, in spite of these successes, still felt there was a vast untouched problem of the 'socially inefficient', which was not being tackled by the law on mental deficiency.

Why were the mentally deficient so important in the scheme of social hygiene? The ideal of social hygiene was a healthy productive workforce and a contented family. It therefore was an actively interventionist philosophy concerned with the 'fit' as much as the unfit. But this vision of the working classes raised to fitness meant a corresponding sorting out and categorisation of the irremediably tainted. This meant the identification among the workforce of the 'unstable' employee, in the family of the 'maternal inefficient' and in society at large of the 'socially inefficient'. Mental deficiency or feeblemindedness was a catchall phrase into which all or most of these categories would fit. Foucault had seen the sciences of social hygiene as sciences of the body and of the individual and to some extent they were. But they were also sciences of very broad social categorisation. This aspect of mental deficiency reached its apotheosis in the Wood Report. This was the report of the Inter-departmental Committee on Mental Deficiency which was published in 1929. The committee had been appointed in 1924 to inquire into the operation of mental deficiency legislation and to survey the extent of mental deficiency in England and Wales. Several members of the Eugenics Society served on it, Evelyn Fox, Burt, Tredgold, F.C. Shrub-sall and Mrs Hume Pinsent. The committee's investigator and resear-cher was E.O. Lewis, who was also a member of the Society.[55] This report was a far greater triumph for the Eugenics Society than anything preceding or following it. This was partly because Lewis's investiga-tion of the incidence of mental deficiency turned up an apparent increase in the problem since 1908 when the last investigation was done under the auspices of the Royal Commission on the Care and Control of the Feebleminded. This alarming fact gave an impetus to eugenic agitation on the dangers of the differential birthrate, the fertility of the inefficient and the need for additional means of control like sterilisation.

Lewis recorded an increase of mental deficiency from 4.6 persons in every 1,000 people in 1908, to 8.56 per 1,000 in 1928.[56] This led to much comment on the doubling of the mentally deficient section of the population since 1908. The Committee was prepared to put down a margin of this increase to Lewis's more rigorous ascertainment. For example, he relied, as in 1908, on returns from institutions, prisons, poor law officers, etc., but he also conducted his own survey of a sample of school children referred to him by teachers as feebleminded, using mental tests. A greater consciousness of the problem among officials might also have led to inflated returns. But the Committee refused to place the burden of the figures entirely on these factors. They emphasised that there had been a real increase.[57]

This would have alarmed the proponents of mental deficiency policy anyway. But Lewis went further. Observing that mental deficients of the higher grade sprang from families of low intelligence but not necessarily themselves certifiable as mentally deficient, he put forward the idea that behind the 300,000 people actually certifiable as mentally deficient according to his estimates, existed much bigger groups of relatives whom he called the sub-cultural or social problem group.

Lewis put a figure of four million or approximately 10 per cent of the population on this group. Moreover, this was a fact of startling social importance for eugenics.

> If, as there is reason to think, mental deficiency, much physical inefficiency, chronic pauperism, recidivism, are all more or less closely related and are all parts of a single focal problem, can it be that poor mental endowment manifesting itself in an incapacity for social adjustment and inability to manage one's affairs, may not be merely a symptom but rather the chief cause of these kindred social evils? If so, then, the problem of mental inefficiency of which mental deficiency is an important part, assumes a yet wider and deeper significance and must indeed be one of the major social problems which a civilised community may be called upon to solve.[58]

As for very low grade mental deficiency, the Report did not consider it as a social problem in the same way as feeblemindedness. They accepted the basic premisses of A.F. Tredgold, who had been an expert witness before the Royal Commission of 1908 and who also served on the Wood Committee. A pre-Mendelian as far as heredity was concerned, Tredgold regarded most of the lower grades of mental deficiency as due to accident or illness and as non-inheritable. Only feeblemindedness was, in his opinion, definitely and indisputably hereditary. In addition to accepting both Tredgold's and Lewis's evidence, the Committee also accepted that statistically the incidence of low grade deficiency was relatively evenly distributed over the social classes but that 'feeblemindedness' was predominantly an affliction of the lower social groups.[59]

There had never been a clearer picture of the socially 'unfit', by reason of heredity, in any preceding report. The Eugenics Society embraced the Wood Report with enthusiasm. It represented an hereditarian explanation of social problems and its alarmist tone seemed to justify a more drastic mental deficiency policy. Therefore the Eugenics Society, under the impact of the Wood Report, launched a campaign for the voluntary sterilisation of the mentally deficient.

Notes

1. Sir Landsborough Thomson, *Half a Century of Medical Research* (HMSO, London, 1970).

2. H.J. Welch and C.S. Myers, *Ten Years of Industrial Psychology* (Sir Isaac Pitman and Sons, London, 1932).

3. See R. Charles, *The Development of Industrial Relations in Britain, 1911-39* (Hutchinson, London, 1973).

4. See L. Urwick, *The Meaning of Rationalization* (Nisbet and Co., London, 1929). See also *The Economist*, vol. 109 (7 December 1929), p. 1073.

5. See also E.P. Cathcart, *The Human Factor in Industry* (Oxford University Press, Oxford, 1928), pp. 15-16.

6. C.S. Myers, *Business Rationalization* (Pitman and Sons, London, 1932), Chapter 1.

7. C.S. Myers, *Mind and Work* (University of London Press, London, 1920), p. 155.

8. Ibid., p. 177.

9. NIIP Papers, Minute Books, 2/1, 1921-4.

10. Ibid., 1938-44, p. 216.

11. See Government Economic Advisory Committee, Committee on Problems of Rationalization, CAB 58/176, pp. 8-15.

12. F.M. Earle, *Methods of Choosing A Career* (George G. Harrap and Co., London, 1931).

13. *Mind and Work*, pp. 168-9.

14. *The Times*, 13 September 1923.

15. See 'Mental Hygiene', *Lancet*, 13 May 1922, pp. 954-5, and *BMJ*, 13 May 1922, pp. 771-2. One of its aims was 'to study social habits, industrial life and environment of people'. *Lancet*, p. 965.

16. *The Times*, 16 July 1926.

17. Report of the deputation of the People's League of Health to the Minister of Health, Neville Chamberlain, 26 June 1927 (Published by the People's League, London, 1928). Lord Horder introduced the deputation, Col. Lelean and C.S. Myers spoke on the relation between health and industrial efficiency. (All three were members of the Eugenics Society).

18. *The Times*, 25 May 1922.

19. Report of the Deputation of the People's League to Montague Barlow. *BMJ*, 12 August 1922, p. 287.

20. Ibid.

21. See 'Vitamins. A Survey of our present knowledge', *MRC Spec. Rep. Ser.*, no. 167, 1932.

22. 'On the Composition of Dietaries', *MRC Report*, no. 13, 1918.

23. Quoted in J.M. Hamill, 'Diet in Relation to Normal Nutrition', *Public Health Reports*, no. 9, 1921, p. 5.

24. *MRC Report*, no. 13, 1918.

25. E.P. Cathcart, 'The Nutrition of Miners and their Families', *MRC Spec. Rep. Ser.*, no. 87, 1924.

26. N. Paton and L. Findlay, 'Poverty, Nutrition and Growth', *MRC Spec. Rep. Ser.*, no. 101, 1926.

27. Ibid., p. 190.

28. Dame Harriette Chick, 'Study of Rickets in Vienna', *Medical History*, vol. 20, no. 6 (1976), pp. 41-51.

29. See N. Paton, 'Discussion on the Importance of Accessory Food Factors in Feeding Children', Section for the Study of Diseases in Childhood, *Proceedings of the Royal Society of Medicine*, vol. 13, 1920, pp. 77-86. For Findlay see 'The Etiology of Rickets', *BMJ*, 4 July 1908, pp. 13-17 and 'A Review of the work done by the Glasgow School on the Etiology of Rickets', *Lancet*, 29 April 1922, pp. 825-31.

30. L. Findlay and Margaret Ferguson, 'A Study of Social and Economic Factors in the Causation of Rickets', *MRC Spec. Rep. Ser.*, no. 20, 1918.

31. H. Corry Mann, 'Rickets. The Relative Importance of Environment and Diet as Factors in Causation', *MRC Spec. Rep. Ser.*, r.ɔ. 68, 1922.

32. See L. Findlay in A.K. Chalmers, W.A. Brend and L. Findlay, 'The Mortalities

of Birth, Infancy and Childhood', *MRC Spec. Rep. Ser.*, no. 10, 1918.

33. *BMJ*, 2 October 1926, p. 607.

34. *The Times*, 13 January 1925.

35. Edward Mellanby, 'Rickets, Osteomalacia and Tetany', *BMJ*, 15 February 1930, p. 289.

36. Kenneth and Jane Morgan, *Portrait of a Progressive; The Political Career of Christopher, Viscount Addison* (Oxford University Press, Oxford, 1980).

37. P.S. Lelean, *How to Feed the Family* (People's League of Health, undated, c. 1927), p. 6.

38. A.L. Chapman and R. Knight, *Wages and Salaries in the UK, 1920-38* (Cambridge University Press, Cambridge, 1953).

39. E.P. Cathcart and A.M.T. Murray, 'Studies in Nutrition', *MRC Spec. Rep. Ser.*, no. 165, 1932, p. 20.

40. *The Times*, 11 March 1926.

41. Corry Mann, 'Rickets', *MRC Spec. Rep. Ser.*, no. 68, 1922.

42. N. Paton and L. Findlay, 'Poverty, Nutrition and Growth', *MRC Spec. Rep. Ser.*, no. 101, 1926.

43. Ibid., p. 110.

44. Ibid., p. 305.

45. Cathcart and Murray, 'A Study in Nutrition. An Inquiry into the Diet of 154 Families in St Andrews', *MRC Spec. Rep. Ser.*, no. 151, 1931; *idem*, 'Studies in Nutrition', no. 165, 1932.

46. Cathcart and Murray, 'A Study in Nutrition', p. 50.

47. Shepherd Dawson and J.C. McConn, 'Intelligence and Disease', *MRC Spec. Rep. Ser.*, no. 162, 1931, pp. 5-6.

48. Eug/D152, Letter to Blacker (from C.W. Saleeby?) on the subject of the New Health Society, 30 July 1928.

49. 'I noticed that precautions were taken to preserve the high standard of our breeds of horses, dogs, cattle, pigs and even chickens *yet our race of humans was left to chance*, that we allowed our unfit to propagate and that we did not even educate our people scientifically in their youth and adolescence in the biological laws which govern offspring.' Olga Nethersole, *The Inception of the League* (People's League of Health, London, 1920), p. 5.

50. *The Times*, 2 February 1926.

51. See the People's League meeting with the LCC and London Juvenile Court Magistrates, January 1925. Reported in the *Lancet*, 17 January 1925, p. 150. They wanted (a) an amendment of the Children's Act 1908 to recognise encephalitis lethargica; (b) special medical and psychological testing in schools.

52. See the journal, *Mental Hygiene*, and the conference held at the Royal Sanitary Institute Congress, Sheffield, July 1929, reported in the *Lancet*, 27 July 1929, pp. 172-5; the Mental Hygiene Conference in London, October 1929, reported in the *Lancet*, 9 November 1929, pp. 998-1001; Mental Hygiene Second Biennial Conference 1931, reported in the *Lancet*, 6 June 1934, pp. 1272-4; and their contribution to the Conference of Medical Officers of Health, 1929, reported in the *Lancet*, 5 January 1929, pp. 22-4.

53. 'Mental Hygiene', *BMJ*, 13 May 1922, pp. 771-2.

54. See Annual Reports of the CAMW especially 1934, 'The First Twenty-one Years'; also see the Journal, *Mental Welfare* (previously *Studies in Mental Inefficiency*), vol. 1, no. 1, January 1920.

55. Report of the Inter-departmental Committee on Mental Deficiency (Wood Report), 1924-29.

56. Ibid., Part IV, 'Investigation into the Incidence of Mental Deficiency in Six Areas', 1925-7, by E.O. Lewis, MA.

57. Ibid., p. 82.

58. Ibid., p. 83.

59. Ibid., p. 135.

5 THE SOCIAL PROBLEM GROUP

> What kind of man is the pauper? What are his antecedents? And what
> are his children likely to become?
> (E.J. Lidbetter, *Eugenics Review*, vol. 11, 1910, p. 169.)

In a memorandum written for the Eugenics Society in 1931, C.P. Blacker,
the incoming secretary, drew up a list of the achievements of the Society
since its foundation in 1907. They had secured the passing of the Mental
Deficiency Act of 1913 and the Amendment to that Act in 1927. By agitation and petition they had helped to get income tax rebates for children.
They had got the Board of Education to put biology into the school cur-
riculum. In the census of 1911 they had had a question inserted on
occupational status, thus enabling demographers to keep track of the
differential birth rate. The remaining major unfinished work was,
according to Blacker, the legalisation of voluntary sterilisation by Act
of Parliament and to that end the Eugenics Society devoted a great deal
of its time in the 1930s.[1]

The issue of sterilisation of the mentally deficient was raised prior
to the 1913 Act. But although some individuals working in the field of
mental deficiency were in favour, others were not. The Royal Commission on the Care and Control of the Feebleminded in 1908 reported that
only 3 out of 21 witnesses who mentioned sterilisation as a solution to
mental deficiency spoke in its favour.[2] In 1922, the CAMW, in
response to a series of articles in *The Morning Post* on 'The Purity of
our Race', canvassed some of its leading experts on mental deficiency
about sterilisation. Of these only Archdall Reid was unequivocally in
favour. A.F. Tredgold admitted its efficacy in a limited number of cases
but, like the majority, was opposed to its legal enactment. In 1923 the
CAMW came out officially against sterilisation and in favour of segregation and institutionalisation as the best means of preventing the propagation of the unfit.[3]

Several things caused reluctance to support sterilisation. First, what
was the legal status of the operation? The Eugenics Society was particularly concerned about this question and it was part of the reason why
they sought an Act of Parliament to clarify the issue. The medical profession feared the operation could result in an action for damages or even
criminal prosecution for assault. When, in the 1930s, the geneticist J.B.S.
Haldane attacked the sterilisation of women as particularly risky and

dangerous these fears must have increased.[4] A second important consideration among followers of social hygiene was the fear that the sterilised mental deficient let loose on the community might spread other 'racial poisons' such as syphilis or behave in an anti-social or unstable manner. Many social hygienists believed that sterilisation might be used as an alternative to institutionalisation and they could not agree with this. Third, what was the state of public opinion on this question? Havelock Ellis advised the Eugenics Society against launching a public campaign or attempting to legalise sterilisation by Act of Parliament.[5] He believed this would only lead to a mobilisation against it by its opponents. The best way to encourage sterilisation was to proselyetise among physicians and to get them to accept it as part of normal therapeutic practice. By doing this, one could simply circumvent the question of its legality.

The Eugenics Society rejected his advice. They saw the Wood Report of 1929 as a vindication of their views on the increasing social cost of mental deficiency and the need for drastic action. This report gave renewed impetus to their campaign. The *BMJ*, for example, prior to 1929 had been sceptical, even hostile, to sterilisation, but on the publication of the Wood Report, whilst not conceding the case for sterilisation, it now believed that a Royal Commission on the subject was 'even more urgently needed than had before been generally realized'.[6] To drive home the conclusions of the Wood Report about the 'social problem group' the *Eugenics Review* in its 1929 October issue announced the formation of a Social Problem Group Investigation Committee to examine the connections this social category had with mental disease and defect, epilepsy, criminality, slums, unemployment, prostitution, inebriety and vagrancy.[7] After the announcement in June 1932 of an inter-departmental committee to examine the question of sterilisation, Blacker tried to steer them towards commitment to this concept. He was in close touch with Lawrence Brock, chairman of the committee, and on 29 August 1933 wrote to him,

> It has therefore occurred to us that there would be no more effective way of organizing further research of this group (social problem group) than that your committee should, in its final report, recommend a detailed inquiry into it. The first volume of Mr E.J. Lidbetter's book is about to appear late this year. It should, in fact, synchronize fairly closely with the publication of your report.[8]

E.J. Lidbetter's list of pauper pedigrees showing the familial incidence of poverty had been begun very early on in the history of the eugenics movement. His research had been aired from time to time in the *Eugenics Review* but the completed study came out in 1933.[9] Four years later, the results of the Eugenics Society Social Problem Group Investigation Committee were published in *A Social Problem Group?* edited by Blacker.[10] The insertion of a question mark after the title is indicative of the feeling that, in an age of mass unemployment and economic depression, some of Lidbetter's conclusions looked distinctly old-fashioned. Blacker became increasingly wary of putting Lidbetter's book forward as the views of the Society, although he remained convinced of its value. A more modern approach to the concept, however, appeared in the work of the demographer Carr Saunders and the sociologist Caradog Jones. These two were members of the Eugenics Society and closely involved with its affairs. Carr Saunders wrote about the demographic and sociological implications of the Wood Report in the *Journal of Mental Welfare* in 1929.[11] He accepted all its significant propositions except that which considered that rural areas had a higher rate of mental deficiency. As a proponent of ruralisation, he found that hard to accept. Similarly Caradog Jones's *Social Survey of Merseyside*,[12] begun in 1929 and published in 1934, was explicitly intended as a further elucidation of the relationship between low intelligence and social problems. Nor did Caradog Jones mince words about the causes of this phenomenon or about the disastrous consequences of indiscriminate social welfare.

> Most of us in these days believe in the principle underlying the social services and we realize the benefits which they have brought the working classes; but I think the time has come when one must exercise more refined methods in selecting those families which are to enjoy these benefits. No humane person would wish to see anybody destitute; but we cannot afford to give and, indeed, we do not at present give without reasonable inquiry into the means of qualifications of applicants for assistance. In particular, those who have any regard for the future of the race will agree that we should try to put a premium on the prevention of a pauper class.[13]

Caradog Jones went on to suggest voluntary sterilisation for the mentally deficient, sexual offenders, criminal recidivists, and feebleminded mothers of illegitimate babies.

The Eugenics Society rested the social case for sterilisation on these grounds and there was in fact a good deal of sympathy for them at government level. Neville Chamberlain, in reply to a deputation in favour of sterilisation from the Grand Council of the National Citizen's Union and the Ladies of the New Health Society, stated,

> . . . I am myself of the opinion that the time is coming when this question of sterilization of the mentally deficient will have to be very seriously considered. . . . It has seemed to me repugnant to common sense that, if a mentally deficient parent or parents on the average, produces or produce similar children the state should allow him to continue to do so . . .[14]

Nevertheless, as the Ministry of Health emphasised both in 1929 and 1935, whilst the policy of sterilisation remained morally controversial and religious authorities in particular were divided, the Government would not put its weight behind it. This was the case regardless of the favourable report given to voluntary sterilisation by the Brock Report in 1934 which came down in favour of legalising voluntary sterilisation.[15]

Moreover the lack of unanimity among the medical profession must have given the government pause for thought. In the BMA the campaign for sterilisation had some notable opponents. The BMA's own report on mental deficiency in 1931 was much more cautious about the causes of it and what could be done about it than the Eugenics Society. In particular, Sir Henry Brackenbury, member of the General Medical Council and of the advisory committee to the Ministry of Health, was a steadfast opponent of sterilisation. It was his opposition and that of Dr Laetitia Fairfield, a Roman Catholic, which prevented the CAMW from reversing its position on sterilisation until 1934 when these two departed from the executive.

There were many points which worried the medical profession. Sir Henry felt sterilisation would put doctors into an exposed social and political position. In addition, the increasing use of the mental test as a diagnostic tool, for example by Lewis in the Wood Report, worried others. On the admission of psychologists, test scores were variable and could be altered by coaching. Since scores followed a curve of normal distribution and only shaded off imperceptibly at the lower end into mental deficiency, it seemed to require an extremely fine sense of judgment to use it to categorise an individual as feebleminded. True, mental deficiency experts accepted that social inefficiency, not test scores, must ultimately be the criterion for certification, but this term 'social inefficiency' or 'incapacity' was itself fraught with difficulties. There was often, some doctors thought, a thin line between the normal life and the socially inefficient one. Who was to say what circumstances might throw an individual into the kind of difficulties indicated by that term? In the end, the diagnosis of higher grade mental deficiency still depended on the impression of dullness of mind given by those who had fallen into social difficulties. But was this sufficient grounds for sterilisation? Moreover, clear evidence of the inheritability of low intelligence was lacking. It ran in families. But so did rickets. Also, the poorer and less protected the family, the more often its members ran the risk of institutionalisation. How could any hard and fast conclusions be drawn about the social incidence of feeblemindedness in these circumstances? Nor was it universally accepted that intrinsic faculty rather than extraneous circumstance was the cause of poverty, crime and illegitimacy.

In addition, what sense did it make to talk of the consent of the higher grade mental deficient to the operation? If the choice was institutionalisation or sterilisation, what value did consent have in these circumstances? Or why should a feebleminded person be presumed to be able to give consent to an operation with such profound consequences whilst, at the same time, considered so incapable of managing their affairs that they could be compulsorily detained? Thus in spite of the favourable report given by Brock in 1934, opinion remained divided.

If the diagnostic and ethical dilemmas presented by sterilisation were difficult, so too were the scientific ones.[16] By 1929, when the debate on sterilisation got under way in Britain, the science of genetics was established at a theoretical and experimental level but knowledge of it in the medical profession and among mental deficiency experts was sketchy if it existed at all. Genetics was not part of medical syllabi. The CAMW lecturers on mental deficiency tended to be people like W.A. Potts and A.F. Tredgold who were educated when genetics was an infant science whose conclusions were hotly contested. Among the general public knowledge was even more limited. The problem was even greater in the application of Mendelian genetics to mental deficiency. Gradually over the 1920s and 1930s studies were published which demonstrated that certain conditions of very severe mental deficiency followed Mendel's laws; that is the chances of inheritance followed the mathematical formulae of Mendel and the conditions exhibited the character of dominance or recession and, in some cases, sex linkage.[17] The Brock Report of 1934 listed some of these studies. So did successive editions of Tredgold's 1908 textbook on Mental Deficiency. But this by no means indicated that mental deficiency experts were by 1934 converted to Mendelism.

One prominent and famous geneticist R.A. Fisher believed, however, that genetics and the mental deficiency policy of the Eugenics Society, including its proposals for sterilisation, were compatible. Fisher had been secretary of the Eugenics Society in the 1920s and, in the 1930s, remained an influential member. He was also an advocate of sterilisation and served on the Brock Committee.[18] Fisher had been attacked in 1917 by R.C. Punnett, another prominent geneticist, for assuming that sterilisation could make any significant impact on the incidence of feeblemindedness. In contrast to Fisher's optimism about sterilisation, Punnett argued that if mental deficiency was a recessive gene, as many then assumed, it would continue to survive in carriers masked by dominant normal genes and its eradication would be excessively long and protracted.[19] Moreover, other geneticists such as J.B.S. Haldane pointed out that if feeblemindedness was a spontaneously occurring mutation, the chances of its eradication were altogether negligible.[20] In any case investigation had revealed by 1930 that feeblemindedness was not a recessive gene and whilst some forms of lower grade mental deficiency were being identified as following Mendelian laws, this was certainly still not the case with feeblemindedness.[21]

Fisher attempted to meet these objections in a number of ways. First, he argued, in opposition to Punnett, that the value of sterilisation would increase if assortive mating — that is the tendency of people with a similar genetic endowment to marry each other — concentrated defect in a certain section of the population. The concentration of higher grade mental deficiency in the lower social classes seemed to indicate that this in fact would happen.[22] Second, he argued that not one but a number of genes might be responsible for feeblemindedness. He called it a multifactorial characteristic dependent upon a number of interacting genetic influences. He also pointed out that, as in other cases of Mendelian inheritance, individuals heterozygous for a characteristic (that is with a mixture of different genes influencing a characteristic) produced intermediate features. This would explain why the higher grade mental deficient seemed to spring from a dull but not mentally deficient section of the population. This concept was taken up by E.O. Lewis, to explain the family relationship between the subcultural social problem group — heterozygous for mental deficiency — and the mental deficients themselves — homozygous (with uniform genes) for mental deficiency.[23]

But Fisher's influence was not the paramount one. Although he served on the Brock Committee and the report of that committee mentioned some conditions of severe mental defect which followed Mendelian laws, the chief influence on them as to the causes of mental deficiency was that of A.F. Tredgold. Tredgold had given evidence to the Royal Commission on the Care and Control of the Feebleminded in 1906-8. His text book *Mental Deficiency* went into eight editions between 1908 and 1952. Although he made some modifications in the light of Mendelian discoveries about mental deficiency in successive editions of this book, his theory of causation was essentially pre-Mendelian.[24] He believed that mental deficiency was an arrest of normal development due to impairment of the germ plasm probably as the result of 'racial poison', whether alcoholism, syphilis or whatever, in past generations. More important his division of mental deficiency into primary amentia and secondary amentia dominated both the Wood Report of 1929 and the Brock Report of 1934. Into the category of primary amentia he put high grade mental deficiency or feeblemindedness. This he considered an hereditary condition as evidenced by low intelligence in the families of mental deficients and sometimes several certifiable mental deficients in the same family. Secondary amentia consisted of most, though not all, of the severe kinds of mental defects. This condition he considered to be environmental, caused by birth injury, pre- and post-natal disease, maternal or childhood illness. As he was not looking for evidence of Mendelian inheritance, the frequent absence of severe mental defect in sibs or near relations of afflicted people or of impairment of intelligence in general among the families of the severely mentally deficient, led him to believe these conditions were not inherited.

Moreover, Tredgold was also a firm believer in the social problem group. In most of his text books he included a passage on the virtues of economic individualism and racial progress. In 1937 he wrote,

> With regard to slums, the trend of evidence is to the effect that these are the result rather than the cause of mental incapacity. . . . I think that if we consider the evidence impartially, and try to divest ourselves of false sentiment and political bias, it will be clear that if it were possible to check the propagation of these markedly psychopathic and inefficient stocks, there would result an appreciable dimunition, not only in the incidence of mental defect, but also in that of many other undesirable conditions which are now a drag upon biological and social advance.[25]

In the last edition of his text book published in 1952, Tredgold repeated his belief in the importance for racial and economic progress of controlling the heredity of the 'submerged tenth'.

These social preconceptions were evident to some geneticists drawn into this controversy. Blacker tried to involve the medical geneticist L.S. Penrose in the investigation of the social problem group. L.S. Penrose was, in 1931, engaged in a series of genetic researches into mental deficiency, for the MRC under the direction of F. Douglas Turner of the Royal Eastern Counties Institution. Blacker wrote to Penrose in 1931 about the important challenge to researchers represented by

four million persons (the 10 per cent sub cultural group) in England and Wales who are the purveyors of social inefficiency, prostitution, feeblemindedness and petty crime, the chief architects of slumdom, the most fertile strain in the community. Four million persons forming the dregs of the community and thriving upon it as the mycelium of some fungus thrives upon a healthy vigorous plant. It is difficult to conceive of a more sweeping or socially significant generalization.[26]

Penrose was not impressed. He wrote back that he thought E.O. Lewis's social problem group needed investigating 'particularly as I am not certain as to whether his hypothesis is correct that there exists such a group'.[27] In addition he complained that the effect of the debate on sterilisation was that a number of families 'have got the wind up about sterilisation and prefer to conceal their family histories'.[28] Shortly after this in 1933 Penrose tested E.O. Lewis's suggestion that the subcultural group was heterozygous for mental deficiency, but no clear confirmatory pattern emerged from these investigations.[29]

Penrose was, meanwhile, commissioned to write a book on mental deficiency by Hogben as part of the series emanating from the latter's department of social biology at the London School of Economics. In this book, *Mental Defect* (1933), Penrose attacked most of the suppositions on which the debate was being conducted.[30] The mentally deficient were not a danger to society, heredity could not be blamed for the variety of social problems mentioned in connection with the social problem group, and cultural deficiency was not a problem of the lower social orders exclusively. Finally, Penrose contended, the laws governing the origin of feeblemindedness were not sufficiently known to justify the sterilisation of the feebleminded.

Penrose's attack upon the Eugenics Society's campaign is paralleled by that of J.B.S. Haldane. In 1934 he launched an attack against the Brock Report in a series of public lectures.[31] In these he disputed the conclusions of the Brock Report that sterilisation would be of value in dealing with the feebleminded. Haldane claimed that it only had value in cases conclusively proved to be due to genetic defect and where those afflicted desired it. These conditions included blue sclerosis or brittle bones, epiloia or lobster claw and some kinds of cataract. But they did not include many conditions of mental defect and certainly not feeblemindedness. Even when a mental defect could be shown to be genetic, sterilisation might be of no use. There were cases where the condition appeared after the end of the reproductive age or by spontaneous mutation. Haldane also insisted that the term 'innate ability' had little meaning given the social determination of what we consider ability to be. This applied particularly to the so-called social problem group.

> There is evidence that their behaviour is partly due to inherited disposi-
> tions, and it is assumed that they would be socially inadequate in other
> environments, as they are in slums. I think this far from certain.
> . . . It is only when people have failed in a favourable environment
> such as we may hope to see throughout Britain in the future that they
> can be regarded as probably unsuitable parents of future generations.
> Differences within a social class are far more likely to be heritable
> than differences between members of distinct classes.[32]

Haldane had raised these doubts in 1933 in a broadcast for the British Broadcasting Corporation in which he crossed swords with J.R. Baker, the friend and colleague of C.P. Blacker. He reiterated them in 1934 and in 1938 brought together his writings and lectures on this subject in a book *Heredity and Politics*. Between 1932, when Haldane publish-ed a book *The Inequality of Man* drawing on his writings in the late 1920s and the publication of *Heredity and Politics* in 1938, Haldane's views had undergone a considerable shift. In the 1920s he had been a propo-nent of scientific rationalism and, just before the First World War, a member of the Eugenics Society. In *The Inequality of Man* in 1932, he proclaimed his aloofness from social systems, 'I cannot accept American and Communist ideals because they are too exclusively economic. They agree in taking economic efficiency to be the principal human virtue. . . . They are both moving towards the mechanisation of life and stan-dardisation of man.'[33] By 1934, however, he was much more sympathetic to Soviet Communism and his views were strongly anti-capitalist. He was also much more strongly anti-eugenic. Haldane, according to the Eugenics Society, was the most intractable opponent of eugenics in this decade. Whilst Hogben was an erratic and increas-ingly hostile ally, Haldane was *persona non grata*.[34] That Haldane's views hit home and had some influence among the working class public was emphasised by the reception afforded to a Eugenics Society public speaker in 1939. Talking to an audience she described as 'well educated working class,' she referred to

> One man in particular, who was in opposition, quoted Haldane's text book in which he says we do not know enough about heredity and . . . that sterilization would be quite useless, also that one third of all London deaths were in the poorhouse and from what I had said they were mentally deficient. A violent environmentalist said that all diseases and defects were produced by bad conditions. I stumped him by mentioning the defects of the well to do classes.[35]

Penrose continued his investigations at the Royal Eastern Counties Institution, finally publishing, in 1938, the Medical Research Council Report number 229 or the Colchester Report as it was known.[36] In this he assembled, from a wide range of sources, the mounting evidence that many forms of severe mental deficiency were inherited according to Mendelian laws. At the same time as he began his investigations for the MRC, a second examination of the causes of mental deficiency was begun under the direction of the Burden Trust. This trust gave financial support to J.A. Fraser Roberts and R.J.A. Berry, both members of the Eugenics Society, to examine mental defectives at the Stoke Park Colony near Bath and to compare them with a sample of the normal population in the City of Bath itself.[37] This investigation was on more traditional lines. It involved the collection of a museum of defective and normal brains (123 defective, 82 normal) for weighing and examination. In addition, it conducted mental tests and sociological studies on the two populations — normal and defective — which were selected for the study. In particular, it tested for the correlation between IQ and family size, maternal age, health, social conditions of the home and occupation. This form of sociological investigation had become a classic tool of the school of 'maternal inefficiency' and, in fact, the study reported its debt to Shepherd Dawson who, apparently, had sketched out the procedures followed. The conclusions of the report, published in February 1938, were that higher grade mental deficiency sprang from a subcultural group among whom social problems were acute and that these social problems were the function of inferior faculty. It also insisted that mental deficiency was a serious and threatening problem.

Almost simultaneously in January of that year, Penrose published his report. It was discussed in July by a group of interested medical men.[38]

The effects of the Colchester Report were considerable. First, the evidence assembled by Penrose destroyed the division between secondary and primary amentia erected by Tredgold. Lower grade mental deficiency could no longer be treated as solely due to environment since many of the cases put by Tredgold into that category were shown to follow Mendelian laws of inheritance. The Report concluded that research should, in future, concentrate on looking at mental defect to see if it followed Mendelian laws. The Report stated that feeblemindedness had still not shown a Mendelian character. It ran in families and that was all. Its causes remained as complex as ever. At the discussion, E.O. Lewis felt that:

> After reading Dr Penrose's report he had the feeling that none of them who were not experts should ever use the word 'heredity.' That word had better be left to the geneticists in future and most of them could not claim an expert knowledge of genetics. Instead of 'heredity' he would suggest some such term as 'familial concentration'. Dr Penrose in his criticism had implied that he (Dr Lewis) had been guilty of using the term heredity rather rashly but he was sure that there were few members present who had not been guilty of the same offence. . . . He thought that for the next decade or so in view of the results of Dr Penrose's researchers they had better confine themselves to looking for genetically typical groups among the lower grade cases.[39]

The *BMJ* felt that the Colchester Report was damaging to the eugenic case. It had never viewed the sterilisation campaign favourably and, in 1938, commenting on the eight years preceding the Colchester Report it claimed:

> Yet throughout this period of time, even in some circles which would claim to be scientific — to say nothing of a wider public more or less interested in social questions — there has been but little dimunition of that uninformed and facile thought, talk and writing which was so prevalent at its beginning. Even today there is a demand for drastic action with regard to mentally defective persons based upon contentions which successive investigations are showing to be false and upon naive explanations of facts which research shows to be far from simple.[40]

None the less the failure of the Eugenics Society's campaign on sterilisation cannot be attributed solely to developments in the science of genetics. In a memorandum for the Society written by Blacker and Cecil Binney in 1956 they attributed the defeat of the campaign to the effect of

Naziism and the opposition of the Roman Catholic Church and the Labour movement.[41] The Labour movement was, they claimed, even more opposed in 1939 than in 1934.

Looking critically at these explanations, the Eugenics Society probably exaggerated the impact of the Nazi Sterilisation Law of 1933. The impact of Naziism on the eugenics movement was much more important in the 1940s than in the 1930s. Certainly, the 1934 Nazi Sterilisation Law embarrassed the Society but not because of its measures, for which there was considerable support in the Society. However, they considered that the compulsory nature of the Act and the political extremism and disruption which accompanied its passing would alienate a section of public opinion.

As for the Roman Catholic Church, there was pretty unanimous condemnation of the campaign for sterilisation from that quarter. Several Catholic MPs were active in securing defeat for the Sterilisation Bill introduced into Parliament in 1931. The Eugenics Society had considerable success in securing support for voluntary sterilisation from other religious groups but if, as the Government claimed, it was not feasible to proceed without the support of 'moral and religious' authorities, then the opposition of the Roman Catholic Church must have been important. Overall the inability of the Eugenics Society to achieve broad consensus across political parties and religious groups accounts for the obduracy of the government in refusing to lend support to a sterilisation bill. In this respect the rise of the Labour Party as the major opposition party in the inter-war years — the 1931 Voluntary Sterilisation Bill introduced privately into Parliament was defeated by their votes — is crucial.[42]

The Eugenics Society were hoist on their own petard. They had won a tremendous success in securing the passing of the Mental Deficiency Bill in 1913 precisely by associating mental deficiency policy with general social and political issues. They had helped to create a 'moral panic'. Perhaps they were perspicacious in believing that legislation of this kind never succeeds or fails on purely scientific grounds. They hoped the Wood Report would create the same kind of moral stampede evident in 1913, and to some extent, it did. However, by the 1930s the political complexion of Parliament and the nation was very different.

The support for sterilisation mobilised by the Eugenics Society in the 1930s was similar to that for the Mental Deficiency Bill of 1913. First were the social hygienists of various hues. Both the CAMW and the National Council for Mental Hygiene were officially represented on the Joint Committee for Sterilisation set up by the Eugenics Society in 1934 to carry on the campaign. So was the Mental Hospitals' Association comprising representatives of the boards of governors of approved institutions for mental deficients. The close links between the Eugenics Movement and social hygiene paid off. All three official representatives of the CAMW on this committee were also members of the Eugenics Society (Evelyn Fox, Cooke-Hurle, and Tredgold) and so were the two from the National Council for Mental Hygiene (R.D. Gillespie and E.W. Neil Hobhouse). Representatives of the New Health Society were prominent in the campaign. Sir William Arbuthnot Lane was signatory to a letter to the *Daily Mail*, 21 February 1929, in favour of sterilisation, and the 'Ladies of the New Health Society' appended their names to a petition in favour, sent to the Ministry of Health in February 1929.[43] Luminaries from the People's League were also important. These included, from the medical council of the People's League, Sir Bruce Bruce-Porter, Sir Farquahar Buzzard, John S. Fairbairn, Alfred Fripp, R.C. Jewesbury, James Purves Stewart and, from the lay side, Lady Melchett, W.A. Appleton, Sir Arthur Yapp and the Honourable Sir Arthur Stanley. Individuals prominent in the Institute for Industrial Psychology also played a part. E.P. Cathcart, Sherrington, Sir Lynden Macassey and Winifred Cullis signed the petition presented to the Ministry of Health and a letter in support of sterilisation to *The Times*, 3 February 1927, was signed by C.S. Myers and Spearman.

Where the precepts of social hygiene had taken root the Eugenics Society was successful in drumming up support for its sterilisation campaign. The Mental Hospitals Association came out in support. So too did the local mental deficiency committees who operated under the aegis of the CAMW to ascertain mental deficiency in an area and to provide guardianship for the mentally deficient. Several organisations connected with the blind were favourably inclined. Local colleges of nursing and midwives' organisations were prominent in registering approval. Although the BMA baulked at sterilisation, the prestigious Royal College of Physicians supported it. The Society of Medical Officers of Health and the Association of County Medical Officers of Health came out in support.[44]

In addition to these medical and quasi-medical organisations, institutions concerned with social work, poor relief and law and order, such as the Magistrates Association, the Insurance Committees (which oversaw the administration of sick benefits) and, in 1929 before its demise, the Association of Poor Law Unions were generally in favour. So was a broad stratum of local government including the County Councils Association and the Association of Municipal Corporations. A major component of support came from women's organisations, namely the National Council for Equal Citizenship, Local Women's Citizens Associations and Townswomen's Guilds.

Looking more closely at this support several things emerge. First, it is almost wholly middle-class. This comes out in the support from local government. Only one elected local government with a Labour majority — Norwich — supported sterilisation. The remainder were Conservative or Liberal, although it is also true to say that not all Conservative or Liberal councils supported sterilisation. However support was likely to be southern and rural. In northern urban areas there was uninterest or even hostility and this reflected the influence of Labour in these areas.[45] In 1934, for example, London which had been in many aspects of its administration a stronghold of social hygiene became a Labour council for the first time in its history. In that year the campaign for sterilisation was in full swing. A motion in support was passed by the local mental hospitals committee but when it was referred to the council itself it was defeated by 63 votes to 44. Most of the opposition came from the Labour members including Herbert Morrison.[46] As Labour recovered from the electoral setback of 1931, and as this recovery was reflected in local government, then the prospect of gaining local political support for sterilisation receded.

The nature of Conservative interest in sterilisation can be gauged from a letter written to the Eugenics Society by the Conservative MP, Wing-Commander James, in 1925,

> Yesterday at the Conservative Conference at Brighton, one Commander Bayley in supporting a resolution upon emigration broke out in what was intended to (be) a eugenic tirade. The substance of his remarks was entirely uninstructed but its reception by some 2,500 representative delegates astonished me. . . . After a reference to breeding from the wrong end of the population (cheers) he advocated a certificate of fitness before marriage (loud cheers) and for the production of children by unlicenced children (*sic*) the penalty of sterilization (loud cheers).[47]

The sentiments expressed at the Conservative Party Conference led James to hope for a breakthrough for the gospel of eugenics. But the very things which helped mobilise this support alienated the Labour Movement. In 1929 the Ministry of Health received two critical memoranda on sterilisation, one from the Birmingham branch of the Distributivist League which was influenced by G.K. Chesterton's social philosophy, and the other from the Public Health Advisory Committee of the Labour Party's Research Division. This stated that

> there is a popular belief that the biologists are in possession of a great body of exact knowledge concerning the transmission of diseases and deficiency which only sentimental or religious prejudice prevents being put to practical use. This is a complete delusion.

The memorandum went on to argue that only a small proportion of mental deficiency was due to heredity. In addition, sterilisation 'would in practice only be applied to the poor'.[48] George Gibson, general secretary of the Mental Hospital Workers' Union, also campaigned vigorously against sterilisation. His union represented non-qualified auxiliary staff in mental hospitals — those who swept, cooked, cleaned, and tended, in non-medical matters, the patients. His members, if they read the *Mental Hospital Workers' Journal*, were extraordinarily well informed on the debate. Their *Journal* covered nearly every major speech or publication on the subject. It also published cartoons which ridiculed the Nazi Law of 1934. Gibson's speeches against sterilisation were singled out by Blacker as particularly noxious. It was due to Gibson's influence that the Trades Union Congress passed a motion against sterilisation in October 1934.

Sterilisation was never a major issue in the Labour movement but where it did impinge upon the consciousness, it was usually received unfavourably. That the working classes should prove so intractable in the realm of negative eugenics is not surprising. Two different social philosophies met head on. A significant section of the Labour movement believed in the social and economic causes of ill-health, unemployment and other family misfortunes and they looked to better and more generous welfare, full employment and a higher standard of living as the solution. If capitalism did not provide this, then so much the worse for capitalism. Social hygiene, in contrast, saw individual 'unfitness' as the cause of social ills. It believed in a better quality of fitness through control of reproduction, the sorting out, quantification and categorisation of the population with a judicious amount of instruction mixed in. If social hygiene was not always favourable to industrial capitalism, it was certainly in favour of property-owning and economic individualism. Economic dislocation was either the individual's own fault (or a product of their innate inferiority), or, if it could be shown to be indisputably the result of the system, it could be dealt with by individual adjustment to the worsened conditions.

This mutual incomprehension was sometimes modified by contact. Miss Hilda Pocock, a Eugenics Society lecturer, who tramped the country in the 1930s spreading the eugenic gospel on its behalf, mainly to women's organisations, rarely reached a male, urban working class audience. But sometimes she did,

> The church is in one of the worst districts of Glasgow. Mrs Whitefield, Secretary of the Secular Society, met me, as she said I had better not wander about there by myself at night. A member of the committee said the people were very red.
>
> The audience, many of whom were unemployed, were very poor and rough, very intelligent and with a keen interest in the slides.
>
> When question time came the chairman had to be very firm and he kept excellent order. . . . As is usual at these meetings the questions were nearly all anti-capitalist and against the present social system and really looking at them one cannot wonder.[49]

When the first Sterilisation Bill was defeated in 1931 by, primarily, Labour votes, C.P. Blacker was conscious of the impression which the Eugenics Society was making among the Left and he was anxious to mitigate it. He wrote to his friend and colleague J.R. Baker, an Oxford biologist, who was about to make a broadcast about eugenics in conjunction with J.B.S. Haldane.

> I have tried to undo the unfavourable impression which has been created by those writers on eugenics who have stressed the question of class. The chief offenders in this direction have been McBride, Dean Inge and our friend Schiller, also Mr Wicksteed Armstrong. . . . If you want the help of the dysgenic you are not very likely to enlist their sympathy if you speak about them as dregs and scum.[50]

Blacker, therefore, advised Baker to moderate his language and stress certain non-controversial aspects of eugenics. However this ploy was not altogether successful for Haldane still attacked Baker in the published transcript of the broadcast. Similarly, Blacker's efforts to mobilise Labour support met with mixed results. In 1935 he set up a National Workers Committee for Sterilisation.[51] Dr Caroline Maule, an unsuccessful Labour candidate in the LCC elections of 1934, was appointed secretary and given a grant of £50 a year to conduct propaganda among the Labour movement. She found it hard going. Outside of Ernest Thurtle, who was also deeply involved in the birth control movement, no prominent Labour parliamentarians were willing to serve on it.[52] Dr Maule could get Labour peers but this was 'inadvisable' in the circumstances.[53] Thus the Workers Committee was thrown back on largely middle-class individuals, a few of whom were members of the LCC.

In addition to this, the Eugenics Society increased its propaganda effort and here they scored a noticeable success. One section of the Labour movement, the Women's Cooperative Guild proved highly receptive and in 1934 their annual conference passed a motion in favour of sterilisation against the tide of opinion in the Labour movement. Miss Pocock, in fact, reported a very favourable reception among the local Women's Cooperative Guilds she approached. Several reasons can be given. The women's section of the Labour movement had revolted against party policy in previous years on the issue of birth control. Many Labour women obviously agreed that any means to control reproduction would, eventually, be of benefit to women.

But it is also clear from the lecturer's reports of these forays into the Women's Cooperative Guild, that the audience frequently felt that, in voting on sterilisation, they were being asked to comment adversely on their more feckless neighbours and their own efficiency and respectability would be judged by their replies. In these circumstances, as the lecturer pointed out, they were often keen to go even further than voluntary sterilisation, advocating its compulsory use. They came out with tales of the scandalous and improvident conduct of persons known to them. Nor can they be blamed for this. Women in families were the target of a great deal of social hygiene propaganda in regard to reproduction, diet and maternal inefficiency. The objective of social hygiene was quite explicitly to convert the mother into the transmission belt for the kind of domestic and child management it thought necessary and virtuous. The effect was profound. What could be more compelling than the thought that your family could starve because of your inefficiency or the idea tha the squalor of your home cold cause your child's rickets? What more appalling than the thought of constant supervision in your home by a lady of better class? Once again the success of eugenics among the Women's Cooperative Guilds was greater in areas of conservative predominance and in the south. The fear of intervention there was greater. The constant complaint of social hygienists of the intractability and inaccessibility of the large industrial city was borne out by their relative lack of success there.

The 1930s saw a leftward movement in opinion among a section of middle-class intellectuals. This had several consequences for social hygiene. It led, for example, to increasing problems for the Eugenics Society. Blacker, the secretary, tried hard to keep middle-class progressives with the Society, particularly those working in the field of heredity. Blacker failed completely with J.B.S. Haldane. He was regarded as no friend to the Society and as a hopeless case. The relations between Penrose and the Society were not easy but Penrose still lectured to them and published his research — even research critical of eugenics — in the *Eugenics Review*. Blacker's relations with others of the same mould were more complex. He found himself, as secretary of the Eugenics Society, conducting a balancing act between the 'old guard' and those whom he described to Baker as 'You, Huxley, Zita and I' who, he believed, represented the progressive core of the Society.[53] Blacker felt that he, in contrast to R.A. Fisher, the previous secretary, represented those in the Society who had a more realistic view of the possibilities of eugenics in the modern world. Thus he regarded his objectives as to lessen exaggeratedly alarmist language, vulgar class prejudice and instinctive suspicion of any scheme involving state intervention. This was not easy. For example, he found it difficult to convince a section of his committee that a scheme for differential family allowances was not creeping socialism.[54] Any modification of the language in which eugenic ideals were expressed in order to mollify his progressive wing was likely to be greeted with suspicion by the 'old guard'.

What and who was this progressive wing? Julian Huxley is a key figure for he was deeply committed to the eugenics movement and involved in its campaign for sterilisation in the 1930s. At the same time he represents 'scientific humanism' and political moderation, though in fact his social views before the radical 1930s, were close to R.A. Fisher's. He was a proponent of modern science and hostile to egalitarianism — a combination quite common in Britain after the First World War. These views came out in a letter he wrote to H.G. Wells in 1930 about a joint literary project in which they were engaged.

As they stand the remarks about different social classes are to me untenable. You make sweeping assertions about the absence of differences between them which I really can't pass. I am quite willing to let you cut out my 'sweeping' assertions about the positive differences between them, but let us point out the problem. To be sure I wasn't biased, I wrote to Carr-Saunders about the point and he writes a long letter back which boils down to what I also had in mind — that the present state of affairs may be eugenically neutral, cannot be eugenically good and probably is slightly eugenically bad.

This concerns the main bulk of the nation. As these differences will I hope soon be wiped out by birth control, I agree to passing it over with a v. slight reference. On the other hand, I have again been reading the Mental Defective Report and it is really quite alarmist (considering what a conservative body the Committee was) about the 'submerged tenth' problem. And this is untouchable by birth control . . . I really think we ought to say something on this point. It comes to this; that the evils of slum life are largely due to the slums, but to a definite extent *caused* by the type of people who, inevitably, gravitate down and will make a slum for themselves if not prevented.[55]

Huxley's interest in scientific humanism brought him a wide circle of friends and contacts with 'progressivism'. The magazine *The Realist* founded by A.G. Church, secretary of the Association of Scientific Workers, member of the Labour Party until 1931, and eugenicist, exemplified the character of twenties' progressivism. The list of supporters and contributors of this magazine is the apotheosis of scientific humanism.[56] But the magazine, like the political ties which held these contributors together, was short lived. Under the impact of economic crisis and European political turmoil, some went to the far left, others to the right. A belief in science, planning and a future without religion was not sufficient to bind together when the questions became planning for what, which science, what non-religious ideologies?

Moreover 'progressivism' and 'left wing' covered a multitude of social attitudes. This is illustrated by Hogben's relationship with the Eugenics Society. Some aspects of his social thought brought him close to the social hygiene movement. First, he disliked industrialisation. He believed in ruralisation, small self-sufficient communities supported by a high level of technology. He believed that socialism should appeal to the salaried white collar stratum rather than to the proletariat.[57] He also believed in a 'healthy national pride' rather than internationalism. He had a brief flirtation with the Next Five Years Group — formed of supporters of the National Government — in 1936.[58] In addition, Hogben considered social hygiene as essential. For example, his writings stressed that the production of children was a social not individual concern and therefore a matter for state control. He thought the control of the quality of the population should devolve upon the expert who he believed was above class or party prejudice. In 1931 he was ambiguous about sterilisation. 'The writer in his capacity as a private citizen does not share the widespread prejudice against voluntary sterilization.'[59] Nor apparently was he opposed to the sterilisation of criminals, the objections to which he saw as specious and sentimental. Thus Huxley counselled Blacker to 'Be patient with H——' when the latter launched a sarcastic attack on eugenics about which Blacker complained.[60]

But the relationship was inevitably stormy. Hogben was a genuine meritocrat and he never considered that the existing social order was a meritocracy. Therefore he favoured equalisation of opportunity and, for all the rhetoric, not one policy promulgated by the Eugenics Society in the 1930s involved an extension of equal opportunity. Hogben's Department of Social Biology in the LSE, meanwhile, engaged in researches to show the environmental component in test scores of intelligence. It sponsored John L. Gray and Pearl Moshinsky's work on the distribution of IQ in the population which demonstrated an untapped pool of ability in the working class which the education system failed to utilise. In addition, the department jointly sponsored with the Eugenics Society a Population Investigation Committee founded in 1935, comprising, among others, the demographers Enid Charles, D.V. Glass and R.R. Kuczynski. The results of this were, largely, above politics as they provided data on which discussions about trends in fertility took place in the late 1930s and 1940s. But individually these three tended to argue for welfare-oriented programmes of social reform to stem the decline in population which agitated so many minds in the late 1930s. Similarly J.L. Gray drew controversial conclusions from his work on the measurement of IQ. For example he disagreed with the research of R.B. Cattell, sponsored by the Eugenics Society, which predicted a decline in national intelligence as the result of differential fertility.[61] Gray had a much more optimistic view about the level of intelligence among the working class. Gray also expressed doubts about the value of the mental test. Finally he criticised eugenics itself.

> Eugenicists have rendered valuable contributions to the study and measurement of mental and physical traits. They dominate the official attitude to the problem of mental defect and influence very largely the common view of the present population crisis. But their theoretical deductions concerning the role of hereditary differences in determining observed differences in human behaviour have recently been subjected to very damaging criticisms, notably by Lancelot Hogben and J.B.S. Haldane. If it is also true that the economic system has gained in recent years a new elasticity, their social recipes will cease to interest us.[62]

These incidents meant that the Eugenics Society's relationship with the Department of Social Biology was never easy. Blacker felt the position with Hogben was the following:

> As long as Darwin and Fisher remain connected with the Society, Hogben would I think, feel a strong temptation to take our money and to guide the research in such a way as to yield conclusions which could be represented as opposed to those which Darwin and Fisher would expect to be yielded. Such a cause would greatly appeal to Hogben's very highly developed sense of humour.[63]

Such an outcome was, in fact, the result of the collaboration between the Social Biology Department and the Eugenics Society.

There were other middle-class radicals who wavered, whilst finally coming down on the anti-sterilisation side. Harold Laski, a pre-1914 eugenicist, who had charmed Pearson himself by his talents and character, still had some residual sympathy with eugenics. (Mrs Laski served on the Workers Committee for Sterilisation.) The trouble was he wanted to have his cake and ha'penny too. The Brock Report, he argued, was 'an admirable document — sane, balanced and clear headed. . . .' On the other hand, it compounded heredity and environment and attributed backwardness due to malnutrition to heredity. But yet, society should protect itself from breeding from stocks 'unquestionably tainted by heredity defects'. On the other hand eugenics too frequently resolves itself into 'class conscious defence of the privileges enjoyed by the rich'. And so on.[64]

As the thirties progressed, Blacker found his political abilities stretched, to keep what remained of the 'progressives' within the Society. This involved him in a good deal of disingenuous comment. Although he complained to Baker about the use of the word 'dregs' it was precisely in these terms that he had written to Penrose two years earlier about the social problem group. Whatever his complaints about the politics of the Nietzschean philosopher, F.C.S. Schiller, Schiller's advice on the strategy to be pursued by the Eugenics Society in the 1930s was exactly that adopted by the Society. Schiller, author of various eugenical tracts,[65] wrote to Blacker on 5 December 1934 advising him, 'to conduct campaigns to popularise the Brock Report, to legalise voluntary sterilisation, to extend the benefits of Birth Control Clinics to the classes which need and desire them most'. Blacker disagreed with none of this, regardless of Schiller's other political views.[66] Blacker wrote to Stella Churchill, a Labour Party member and an enthusiast for the idea of prenuptial health certificates, that 'In my private opinion the essential principles of eugenics harmonise much better with the Socialist Party's conception as to the proper distribution of wealth.'[67] A few years before this he had commended eugenics to the Conservative Party as in accord with its principles and commitments.[68] He also kept up a correspondence with Lord Horder, the President of the Society, critical of the commentaries issuing from Hogben's Social Biology Department.[69] Blacker tried to sooth Huxley's anger at Cattell's book *The Decline of National Intelligence* — a book written under the auspices of the Society.[70] A few years later he was recommending it to W.B. Yeats when the latter wrote asking him for a book-list on differential intelligence.[71] The clue to these contradictions lies in the clear perception Blacker had that the public image of eugenics in the 1930s was, for the first time, doing it harm among some people who had been previously its natural constituency. Blacker pointed out that when the lower 'fitness' and intelligence of the working class was propounded 'It is safe of course to write these things in the sanctity of one's study. But is it safe to say them to audiences of working or unemployed men, in a big industrial centre?'[72] But Blacker's efforts to modernise the Society were largely in the realm of its rhetoric and nomenclature. At the centre of disparate and conflicting tendencies, Blacker felt it his duty to keep them from flying apart. Nevertheless by 1939 the fact that the Eugenics Society had not changed substantially since 1929 was soon to land it in difficulties.

Notes

1. Eug/C27, 7 October 1931.
2. See Report of the Royal Commission on the Care and Control of the Feebleminded (1908) Cmnd 4202.
3. See *Studies in Mental Inefficiency*, vol. 3 (1923). This position held until 1934. See *Annual Report of the CAMW*, 1934-5, p. 21.
4. J.B.S. Haldane, *Human Biology and Politics*. The Tenth Annual Norman Lockyer Lecture, delivered 28 November 1934 at the Goldsmiths Hall (British Science Guild, London, 1935), p. 13. For Haldane see G. Werskey, *The Visible College* (Allen Lane, London, 1978) and Ronald Clark, *JBS* (Hodder and Stoughton Ltd, London, 1968).
5. See 'Havelock Ellis, Obituary', *Eugenics Review*, vol. 31 (July 1939), p. 111.
6. *BMJ*, 27 April 1929, p. 109.
7. B. Mallet, 'The Social Problem Group', *Eugenics Review*, vol. 23 (October 1931), pp. 203-6.
8. Eug/D50, Blacker to Brock, 29 August 1933.
9. E.J. Lidbetter, *Heredity and the Social Problem Group* (E. Arnold and Co., London, 1933).
10. P. Blacker (ed.) *A Social Problem Group?* (Oxford University Press, Oxford, 1937).

11. Carr Saunders, 'Report of the Special Investigation carried out on behalf of the Joint Committee', *Mental Welfare*, vol. 10, no. 2 (1929) pp. 41-6.

12. D. Caradog Jones, *The Social Survey of Merseyside* (Hodder and Stoughton, London, 1934).

13. Eug/C193, Caradog Jones, *Mental Deficiency on Merseyside*. Address to the Annual Conference of Mental Health Workers, 17 April 1932, p. 8.

14. MH58/103, 20 February 1939.

15. MH58/100, 17 May 1935.

16. For an account of the development of genetical science in Britain and elsewhere, see Garland Allen, *Life Science in the Twentieth Century* (Wiley, New York, 1975); Ernst Mayr, *The Growth of Biological Thought* (Belknap Press for Harvard University, Cambridge, Mass., 1982); and R.C. Punnett, 'Early Days of Genetics', *Heredity*, vol. 4, pt 1 (April 1950) pp. 1-10.

17. See Penrose's introduction to *MRC Spec. Rep. Ser.*, no. 229, 1938 in which these studies are listed.

18. For Fisher, see Joan Box, *R.A. Fisher. The Life of a Scientist* (Wiley, New York, 1978); D. MacKenzie, *Statistics in Britain* (Edinburgh University Press, Edinburgh, 1981); B. Norton, 'Fisher and the neo-Darwinist synthesis' in E.G. Forbes (ed.) *The Human Implications of Scientific Advance* (Edinburgh University Press, Edinburgh, 1978).

19. R.C. Punnett, *Journal of Heredity*, vol. 8 (1917) p. 465.

20. Haldane, Tenth Annual Norman Lockyer Lecture, 28 November 1934, reported in MH51/556.

21. See S.P. Davies, *Social Control of the Mentally Deficient* (Constable and Co., London, 1930).

22. R.A. Fisher, 'The Elimination of Mental Defect', *Eugenics Review*, vol. 16 (April 1924) pp. 114-16.

23. E.O. Lewis, 'Mental Deficiency, The Sub Cultural Group', Address to the British Association, 1931 reprinted in *Eugenics Review*, vol. 24 (April-Jan. 1933), p. 289 and *Journal of Mental Science*, vol. 79, (1933) pp. 298-304.

24. A.F. Tredgold, *Mental Deficiency* (Ballière, Tindall and Cox, London, 1908). See also fifth edn., 1929 and sixth edn., 1937.

25. Ibid., sixth edn., 1937, p. 522.

26. Penrose Papers 130/9, Blacker to Penrose, 1 October 1931.

27. Ibid., Penrose to Blacker, 2 October 1931.

28. Ibid.

29. L.S. Penrose, 'Mental Deficiency — II. The Sub Cultural Group', *Eugenics Review*, vol. 24 (January 1933) pp. 289-91.

30. L.S. Penrose, *Mental Defect* (Sidgwick and Jackson, London, 1933).

31. See J.B.S. Haldane, speech at the Central Library, Sheffield, 15 November 1934, and the Tenth Annual Norman Lockyer Lecture, 28 November 1934. Also see J.R. Baker and J.B.S. Haldane, *Biology in Everyday Life* (Allen and Unwin, London, 1933); J.B.S. Haldane, *Heredity and Politics* (Allen and Unwin, London, 1938).

32. J.B.S. Haldane, Tenth Annual Norman Lockyer Lecture, p. 15.

33. J.B.S. Haldane, *The Inequality of Man* (Chatto and Windus, London, 1932), p. 227.

34. Blacker to Mrs Neville Rolfe, 14 February 1935, Eug/D79. 'The difficulty arises of conveying the views of the sub committee of our council to Professor Haldane in a manner that would not annoy him. As you doubtless know he is not at all favourably disposed to this Society and may well regard suggestions emanating from us as an impertinence.'

35. Eug/G13, 'Propaganda and Publicity. Lecturers' Reports', Lecture given by Miss Hilda Pocock of the Eugenics Society at the Glasgow Secular Hall, 12 March 1939 to 250 (20 women) described as well educated working class.

36. L.S. Penrose, 'A Clinical and Genetic Study of 1280 Cases of Mental Defect', *MRC, Spec. Rep. Ser.*, no. 229, 1938.

37. *BMJ*, 18 February 1938, p. 333.

38. See T.A. Munro, 'Discussion on Consanguinity and Mental Disorder', *Journal of Mental Science*, vol. 84 (September 1938), pp. 708-14, 716 (Meeting 6 July 1938).

39. Ibid.

40. 'A Study of Mental Defect. Report by Dr Penrose', *BMJ*, 26 March 1938, pp. 687-9.

41. Eug/C27, 27 June 1956.

42. The 1931 bill was defeated by 167 votes to 89.

43. MH58/103, 16 February 1929.

44. Taken from Eugenics Society List of Resolutions passed in favour of sterilisation, 1934-6.

45. The Parliamentary Committee set up by the Eugenics Society in 1932 to pursue a sterilisation law included four Conservatives, Katherine Atholl, Vyvian Adams, C.T. Culverwell, A. James; two Liberals, George Lambert and William Mabane; and one National Labour MP, Holford Knight.

46. See *The Times*, 4 July 1934.

47. Eug/C190, Letter to Eugenics Society, 9 October 1925.

48. MH58/104A, memo no. 168a.

49. Eug/G13, 'Propaganda and Publicity, Lecturers' Reports', meeting at the Unitarian Church, Ross Street, Glasgow. 120 present (5 women).

50. Eug/C10, Blacker to Baker, 15 February 1933.

51. See Eug/D150, National Workers Committee, 1935-38. On it were Mrs John Wilmot, Mrs Charles Latham, Mrs Harold Laski, Mrs M.E. Stroudley, Mrs Clegg and Dr Eileen Warren. Invited to join were Ruth Darwin, Rev. Belben, Rev. Chesney, C.P. Trevelyan, C. Robertson and Emil Davies.

52. Eug/D150, Caroline Maule to Blacker, 3 October 1935.

53. Ibid.

54. Eug/C108, Blacker to Fisher, 14 December 1933. 'Much of the hostility to family allowances in the council springs from a confusion of ideas about the effects of different schemes of family allowances.'

55. Huxley to H.G. Wells, 10 February 1930. Quoted in J.S. Huxley, *Memories I*, 2nd edn (Allen and Unwin, London, 1970), pp. 168-9.

56. See the editorial board, *The Realist*, vol. I, 1929. This included J.B.S. Haldane, B. Malinowski, Sir Richard Gregory, Carr Saunders, H.J. Laski, Julian and Aldous Huxley, Herbert Read and A.G. Church. The subsequent issues included Myers on Industrial Psychology and Lewis on Mental Deficiency.

57. L. Hogben, *The Retreat from Reason*, Conway Memorial Lecture (Walter and Co., London, 1936), p. 55.

58. See Allen Papers, NFYG, 1936.

59. L. Hogben, *Genetic Principles in Medicine and Social Science* (Williams and Norgate, London, 1931), p. 203.

60. Eug/C185, Blacker to Huxley, 24 October 1930, and Huxley to Blacker, 4 November 1930.

61. See R.B. Cattell, *The Fight for our National Intelligence* (P. & S. King, London, 1937). The results became known earlier and resulted in a public disagreement between Gray and Cattell.

62. J.L. Gray, *The Nation's Intelligence* (Watts and Co., London, 1936), p. 22.

63. Eug/C172, Blacker to Horder, 14 January 1938.

64. *Time and Tide*, 27 June 1934; MG51/56, Press Cuttings.

65. See F.C.S. Schiller, *Social Decay and Eugenical Reform* (Constable and Co., London, 1932).

66. Eug/C309, F.C.S. Schiller to Blacker, 5 December 1934. These tended to be pro-aristocracy. Blacker, however, had far more trouble with another proponent of the radical right, Pitt Rivers, who left the Society in 1932 on the grounds of its lack of radicalism; see Eug/I2.

67. Eug/C68, Blacker to Stella Churchill, 30 April 1931.

68. 'C P B', 'The control of population', three articles for *Saturday Review*, vol. 140 (1925) pp. 11, 40, 69.

69. Eug/C172. Blacker to Horder, 26 March 1937. On Glass's book 'I cannot myself help feeling from the standpoint of a committee (Population Investigation Committee) whose object it is to promote research of an objective scientific character that the book was inappropriately written.'

70. Eug/C64, Huxley to Blacker, 16 April 1937, and Eug/C185, Huxley to Blacker, 9 January 1936.

71. See Eug/C357, Yeats Correspondence.

72. Eug/C57, Memo by Blacker on 'The Formation of an Institute of Family Relations', 11 January 1935, p. 2.

> The Plan will aim at replacing the disorderly existing political and economic system by a reconstituted machine based on the application of science to social and political affairs.
>
> (PEP Papers, WG2, PEP & Publicity, 16 July 1932.)

From 1929 to 1931 the world economic system was badly affected by crisis and depression. Unemployment mounted in most industrial nations. In Britain, by 1933, it had reached three million.[1] In August 1931 the Labour Prime Minister, Ramsay MacDonald, decided to call on all political parties to form a National Government to deal with the economic crisis. He hoped a National Government would have the authority to make substantial cuts in public expenditure, including unemployment pay. A majority of his Labour colleagues disagreed with him and the Labour government resigned. In October 1931 MacDonald called a general election in which a National Coalition of Conservatives, Liberals and some breakaway Labour members was returned with an overwhelming majority. The Labour Party lost a considerable number of seats.[2] MacDonald's support in Parliament and the country was overwhelmingly Conservative and Liberal. A few Labour party members supported his actions and these formed the National Labour Party in 1931.

The crisis of 1931 was to have many effects. Among these was the emergence of a group of intellectuals who believed the failure of Britain's economic system in 1931 could be blamed on the lack of long-term, scientific planning. They saw planning as a means to extricate Britain from her difficulties and they also saw it as something which could draw support from all parties. Typical of these groups were Political and Economic Planning (PEP) and the Next Five Years Group (NFYG).

PEP came into being on the initiative of Max Nicholson and Gerald Barry. In 1930 these two met informally to discuss the need for a National Plan to aid economic recovery. Barry was editor of the periodical *Weekend Review*. He used it in February 1931 to publish a supplement, written by Nicholson, outlining their proposals. They gradually drew around them individuals interested in their ideas and in March 1931 they issued the first public statement outlining the formation of a planning group which became known as PEP. They also appointed a general council to run it. By April 1933 they had established a structure of committees and discussion groups and had published their first broadsheet or

113

discussion document. The source of funding for the group was the ten shillings annual subscription, plus donations from Basil Blackett, Israel Sieff and the trustees of Dartington Hall (a charitable trust engaged in educational and other activities). Kenneth Lindsay, who was a party to the discussions leading to the foundation of PEP, became general secretary and editor of their periodical, *Planning*. By 1935 PEP had to admit that they had failed to produce a National Plan for Britain. But they had established themselves successfully as an independent research and intelligence unit and, as such, they proved remarkably enduring.[3]

Almost simultaneously the Next Five Years Group came into existence. The motivating spirit was Clifford Allen, a former Labour Party politician who had followed Ramsay MacDonald in 1931 into the Coalition government and was now prominent in the National Labour Party. In 1932 he was keen to draw together what he called 'progressive' opinion from all political parties to work out an agreed programme on social, economic and international policy. He drew support from two 'progressive' Conservatives, Harold Macmillan and Hugh Molson, and a variety of Liberal and usually ex-Labour politicians and intellectuals. In February 1934 the NFYG issued a manifesto, *Liberty and Democratic Leadership*. This was a public commitment to democracy and non-violence in politics rather than an economic and social manifesto. In 1935 however they produced a more detailed description of the social and economic developments they favoured in a book entitled *The Next Five Years*. After the publication of this, the NFYG created a number of working committees. From time to time it published blueprints for the future and, for a while, a journal, *New Outlook*, edited by Macmillan and his friends. The NFYG received financial support from various individuals including Hugh Molson, L.J. Cadbury, R.A. Bray, Graham White, Lady Rhondda, Eleanor Rathbone, Seebohm Rowntree and A.L. Hobhouse. Clifford Allen's death in 1938 and the outbreak of the war in 1939 resulted in the break-up of the group. Also the political and economic crisis which had generated the NFYG had by the late 1930s passed and therefore much of the *raison d'être* for the group had disappeared too.

But so had much of the *raison d'être* for PEP which was also seen by its founders as a response to the crisis of 1929-31 but which, none the less, survived into the post-war world. However, there was a difference. The NFYG saw its role as much more directly political. It wanted to intervene in current political controversies by reconstituting a body of moderate or 'middle opinion' drawn from all political parties. PEP, after its failure to produce a National Plan, contented itself with a policy of permeation of existing political parties, modelling its role on that of the

Fabians before 1914. Yet their common emphasis on a detailed, planned response to 1929-31 and on mobilising the unprejudiced, scientifically minded planners across party lines meant there was considerable overlap between the two groups.

The core of PEP in the 1930s was, according to the history written by Kenneth Lindsay, some dozen people. In the early years, Gerald Barry, editor of *Weekend Review* (which merged in 1934 with the *New Statesman*), Basil Blackett and Arthur Salter were prominent. Salter and Blackett were economists and important public officials. Leonard Elmhirst of Dartington Hall, Sir Geoffrey Whiskard, a civil servant, Israel Sieff, director of Marks and Spencer's department stores, Noel Hall, Professor of Economics at University College, Julian Huxley and Sir Henry Bunbury, Controller and Accountant General at the Post Office were also important. To these must be added R.C. Davison an ex civil servant and expert on unemployment, John Dower, an architect, Oliver Roskill, an industrial consultant, and finally the moving spirits of PEP, Max Nicholson and Kenneth Lindsay.

The group in PEP who worked on health and social policy were slightly different. R.C. Davison was an important figure in these fields. From 1934 he served simultaneously on the Employment, Health, Civic, Social Assistance and Social Services committees of PEP. W. Eager of the National Institute for the Blind, E.P. Lascelles, a member of the Royal Commission on Unemployment Insurance and A.D.K. Owen served on the Health, Employment and Civic divisions of PEP. A.D.K. Owen was later released from PEP to work on *Men Without Work* for the Pilgrim Trust, an investigation of the effects of unemployment on the industrial workforce. Carr Saunders, at first relatively inactive, became an important contributor to PEP social policy from 1935. He became chairman of the Social Services Committee in 1937 and a member of the council of PEP in the 1940s.[4]

There was also some interchange of personnel between PEP and NFYG. After an initial skirmish with PEP, Salter became important in the NFYG. Sieff stayed with PEP although the NFYG approached him for help. However, he remained close to Macmillan who was a leading figure in the NFYG. PEP contacts were listed by the NFYG as J.J. Mallon, Hugh Molson and Arthur Salter, and Allen Young, Macmillan's secretary. R.C. Davison was co-opted into the Social Services Committee of the NFYG as was S.S. Metz of PEP and the hard-pressed Julian Huxley was a member of both groups. Eleanor Rathbone served on the NFYG's Social Services Committee performing the same role there as an advocate of family allowances as Eva Hubback, her close friend, did in PEP.

There was an ideological as well as a personal overlap. These two groups, at least in the early 1930s, were apologists for the National Government. Hugh Molson, for example, felt that:

> Few people believe that orthodox Tory doctrines are adapted to post war or, at any rate, post crisis conditions. Few people regard the old fashioned Socialism as a panacea for modern ills. Fewer still are free traders. The National Government offers a means of developing a new policy which will have to cut across old Party programmes and . . . personal prejudices if it is to cope with the new economic conditions.[5]

Similarly Basil Blackett believed that, with the advent of a National Government in 1931, there had been an improvement in the prospects for economic planning. He continued, until his death in 1935, to sing the praises of the National Government.[6]

This support was natural for Conservatives like Molson and Blackett. A good three-quarters of the support for the National Government in Parliament was drawn from the Conservative Party. But the appeal of the National Government was just as significant among the 'Left' of the planning movement. There was a strong group of planners around the National Labour Party, a section which split from the official Labour Party to follow Ramsay MacDonald into the National Government. Clifford Allen of the NFYG was a key figure here. Geoffrey Elton, Herbert Dunnico and R.D. Denman were also members of the NFYG and the National Labour Party. Within PEP, Kenneth Lindsay was National Labour MP for Kilmarnock and a junior minister in MacDonald's government. Due to his contacts some of the PEP's discussions were held under the aegis of MacDonald at Number 10. Oliver Roskill, Noel Hall, R.C. Davison and Alfred Zimmern, an expert in international relations, were also members of the National Labour Party and PEP. The pages of the *National Labour Newsletter* were full of contributions from NFYG and PEP. In addition, in 1934, Lindsay, Davison, Zimmern, Elton and Denman drew up the policy documents for the National Labour Party on social, economic and international questions.[7] The PEP policy for employment 'Exit and Entrance to Industry' bore a strong resemblance to that presented by the National Labour Party.

The epithet 'national' had always had a strong pull on some members of the Labour Movement. C.W. Bowerman, and George N. Barnes re-emerged in the 1930s to join the NFYG recalling an earlier era when the Labour Party produced another 'national' offshoot. The first manifesto of NFYG, which committed its signatories to the defence of democracy and non-violence, was signed by the Labour politicians George Lansbury, Hugh Dalton, Noel Baker and Ernest Bevin. Allen also singled out Tom Johnston, Lee Smith, Noel Buxton and Mary Agnes Hamilton in the Labour Party as sympathetic to the NFYG. However, the Labour Party Chairman, Arthur Greenwood, intervened to put a stop to further contacts and of the Labourists only Arthur Pugh, Henry Brinton and John Bromley remained close to the NFYG. For many it was party discipline which severed the connection. But to others it was the suspicion that, in spite of Allen's pleas that 'this is not a device inspired by the National Government'[8] it was precisely that. PEP, however, even with less overt political content, still drew from largely the same constituency as the NFYG. They too engaged in the rhetoric of national unity, of science as a device to transcend class struggle and planning as politically neutral.

The planning programmes of PEP and the NFYG have to be seen in the context of the relationship of these groups to the National Government. These programmes were suffused with the financial orthodoxy which the National Government in 1931 was pledged to uphold. Of the 37 signatories to the Keynes-inspired letter to *The Times* on 10 March 1933, asking for an expansion of the economy through public works, only four were members of either PEP or the NFYG and of these four only one was an economist, Professor Sargeant Florence.[9] There were strong proponents of public works in PEP and NFYG but they tended to take the position of the *Economist* a leading financial journal, supporting public works and deflation simultaneously.

The *Economist*, for example, in February 1931 attacked the Treasury Memorandum of 1929 which criticised the raising of loans for public works during times of depression. But they also criticised those who saw loans for public works as anything other than relief, whose function was primarily political not economic. They defended the balanced budget and attacked rigidity of wage levels — all very much part of current economic orthodoxy. They insisted that, whilst public works should be on socially useful projects, they should be prevented, as far as possible, from interfering with or having any effect on private industry. Their objective was not reflation but diffusion of the potential social explosiveness of unemployment. Public works, the *Economist* argued, should be abandoned when the economy was on the upturn. They could neither effect this upturn nor sustain it. The *Economist*'s advocacy of public works tended to wane as the likelihood of social turmoil caused by unemployment proved illusory. This fear of social dislocation had encouraged the *Economist* to support the National Government of 1931 in spite of the strong possibility it would introduce tariffs which it vehemently opposed.[10]

What then did it mean to talk of economic planning if not expansion, public works and reflation? The economist Lionel Robbins, an adherent of *laissez-faire* economics, commented on the popularity of the word 'planning' in 1934

> Socialism is a term which is not universally popular. But 'planning' — ah magic word! Who would not plan? We may not all be socialists now, but we are certainly (nearly) all planners. Yet if planning is not a polite name for giving sectional advantages to particular industries, what does it denote but socialism?[11]

The economic planning of PEP and the NFYG was certainly not socialism. Instead it fits Robbins's alternative definition. The planning of PEP and NFYG was rationalisation, the encouragement of industrial amalgamation, the elimination of wasteful competition and control of marketing and production.

Allen Young, Macmillan's secretary, wrote to Clifford Allen in 1933 about the economic policy around which the 'middle way' could be constructed. 'The basis on which agreement might be found,' he argued, 'is in acceptance of the view that capitalism must be pushed into its monopolistic phase.'[12] The encouragement of amalgamation of industry was one of the objectives of the Industrial Reorganisation League founded by Macmillan and Henry Mond (second Lord Melchett and director of Imperial Chemical Industries). This had an executive committee of about 60 businessmen and economists which included Israel Sieff, an important figure in PEP.[13] Clifford Allen wrote approvingly of the League to Macmillan and Macmillan was given the chapters on Industrial Reorganisation for the book, *The Next Five Years*.[14]

Rationalisation gripped PEP even more strongly. They saw it as covering not only amalgamation but also the planning of purchasing and distribution, scientific research, scientific management and the coordination of marketing. It was, they believed, the ultimate solution to the problems of Britain's ailing industries, particularly coal and cotton. PEP believed that the National Government was sympathetic to rationalisation.[15] But both PEP and the Industrial Reorganisation League wanted a more interventionist role on the part of the state. PEP set up a group to consider drawing up a parliamentary bill to encourage amalgamation.[16] Simultaneously, in 1934, the Industrial Reorganisation League, acting through its parliamentary representatives, Hugh Molson and T.B. Martin, tried to get an Enabling Bill, to speed rationalisation, through the House of Commons. The bill in the Commons was, however, dropped. In addition, PEP's interest in permissive legislation faded. On the whole, they could get no large-scale support from industry for these plans. Rationalisation, it was pointed out to them, took place anyway and the legal and political climate in Britain was generally favourable to it. The only legally enforceable right industry wanted was price fixing and neither PEP nor the Industrial Reorganisation League wanted to be associated publicly with that.

This fascination with rationalisation went further than amalgamation, especially in PEP. The large amalgamated firm was seen as having political and social as well as economic functions. First, monopolised industries, overseen by a National Industrial Council, would group employees and employers in self-governing industrial councils in which wages and conditions would be settled jointly. PEP was keen that this self government should extend to social security. They believed that there should be a state-provided minimum to fall back on but that major insurance against sickness and accident should be provided by private industry. This vision of social security, industrial peace and self government was close to corporatism. Molson spoke approvingly of Mussolini's Italian experiment and PEP flirted briefly with Oswald Mosley, the leader of British Fascism.[17]

The relationship of rationalisation to the cure of unemployment, it was argued, was that amalgamations would ultimately smooth out violent fluctuations in the economy and by increasing productivity lead to a general rise in employment. But it was fully admitted that it offered no immediate relief nor was this its function. Nor, so the argument went, could any other form of economic reconstruction. Public works were seen as sources of poor relief and outlets for social frustration.

What had all this to do with social hygiene? A great deal for it formed the framework in which social and health policy was discussed. If a decline in unemployment had to await a general revival in trade what immediate measures for improving the social conditions of the poor were available? They resolved themselves into control and manipulation of the population. This is perfectly expressed in PEP's employment policy, *Exit and Entrance to Industry*. It proposed raising the school leaving age and dropping the age of retirement thus artificially limiting the labour force.[18] In PEP's discussions other measures of this sort were canvassed. One solution — and a favourite of social hygiene — was emigration. But countries suffering from economic depression had ceased to take many immigrants. Getting rid of woman's work was discussed. However, a great many industries relied on the relative cheapness of female labour and this was scotched too. Stopping Irish immigration was also considered but the same objections applied to this.[19] Some industries also traditionally relied on Irish immigration.

All these ideas involved artificial restriction or limitation of the labour force. Logically, therefore, the precepts of social hygiene for limiting the working-class birth rate and eliminating the dysgenic section of the workforce were part and parcel of them. The proponents of rationalisation made this quite clear. Molson, the year before he introduced the Enabling Bill to encourage amalgamations, introduced a bill for voluntary sterilisation into the House of Commons. Mental deficients, he claimed, not only composed the social problem group but, 'it is these stocks which contribute a vast quantity of the unorganised, unskilled, casual labour which is so often upon the rates and which so often undercuts a higher, more skilled type of labour'.[20] Similarly the *Weekend Review*'s proposals for economic planning also included the elimination of the 'dysgenic' and 'the education of a small, highly efficient, healthy labour force in place of the old ragged army'.[21]

The welfare schemes offered by the planning movement were of two sorts. First was the reorganisation and rationalisation of the existing social services. The NFYG described their work on social administration, as 'a study of the existing machinery for social insurance and the administrative savings and increased efficiency which might be secured by the coordination of all the insurance schemes in a single Department of Insurance'.[22] Second, the planning groups wanted the extension of social insurance to parts of the workforce or classes of problem (i.e. accidents) which were still outside its present scope. This was something already accepted by the government in principle but which still had not been fully enacted in practice. The PEP 1937 report on the rationalisation of the British health services put these ideas forward and its comprehensive discussion of the question proved influential. Both groups, however, were strong supporters of the means test — an instrument detested in areas of high unemployment — but strongly defended by Davison, their social affairs expert. The insurance principle — benefit measured by contributions supplemented by non-contributory but means-tested relief — was sacrosanct to PEP and the NFYG. They also played about with a few other ideas for helping the unemployed. Public works for 'socially useful' projects were mentioned by the NFYG along with the provision of rural homesteads as an alternative to industrial employ-ment.[23]

Neither of these groups anticipated the sweeping changes in social welfare brought about by Beveridge in the 1940s. PEP, for example, was totally against a state-run health service preferring a private one with a minimum state provision for the needy and medical insurance schemes run by industries. Similarly, the NFYG regarded an extension of existing medical insurance as the way forward. Nor was there any idea of a national minimum below which the sick, unemployed or employed should not fall. PEP examined the idea of a non-contributory scheme but rejected it, 'the view of this group is that a national scheme providing relief according to need for vast numbers of able bodied who are genuine workers is fundamentally unsound'.[24] Instead they advocated more private employers' insurance schemes against unemployment and, 'an expansion of thrift and provision against misfortune'.[25] Rathbone beavered away in the NFYG to get its support for family allowances but to no avail. 'It was felt (by the committee), however, that any pro-posal for the alteration of the wage system ought properly to come under the consideration of the industrial organization committee.'[26]

These considerations affected the planning movement's attitude to the question of nutrition among the poor which became in the 1930s a sub-ject of intense controversy. The NFYG in its *Programme of Priorities* in 1937 talked of 'scales of unemployment and public assistance to be considered in the light of calculations of subsistence needs by compe-tent scientific and medical authorities'.[27] But it got no further than this rather ambiguous statement. On the whole, given the reluctance of the planning movement to condone raising the level of consumption among the poor, their solution to the problem of inadequate diet was unadventurous.

PEP spent more time discussing the problem. F.R. Cowell was on their nutrition committee and responsible for drawing up memoranda and, eventually, their broadsheets on this question.[28] Also on the nutri-tion committee were Edward Mellanby, Max Nicholson, and Professor A.W. Ashby. In the document he drew up for them, F.R. Cowell refer-red to 'the discoveries made in the last twenty years about nutrition'.[29] His suggestions for improving standards of nutrition were the eradica-tion of bovine TB and cleaner supplies of milk. To this he added free milk to nursing mothers and a greater knowledge of nutrition. At the same time,

Obviously dietary standards cannot be presented without reference to economic factors. If, therefore, society finds itself unable to afford its unemployed the scale of diet necessary to maintain health, it is all the more urgent that the unavoidable damage to the health of the unemployed and their dependants should be reduced to the lowest degree compatible with the state of national poverty of which such a provision will at one be an expression and an index.[30]

This of course was the crucial question. If one accepted 'the state of national poverty' as a restraining factor, what kind of food policy could be offered to these on unemployment pay or low wages? This was a highly controversial question in the mid-1930s.

PEP's nutrition committee answered it by the assumptions of social hygiene. Mellanby believed that 'the [chief] difficulty arises from public ignorance and apathy. The difficulty of converting people to a scientific view of the problem is enormous.'[31] He also lambasted government policy. The distribution of free milk to school children had helped but it had been done to relieve the problems of milk producers by offering them a subsidy not as part of a concerted campaign on health. Nicholson repeated the idea that 'the real problem was publicity'.[32] This would be a major aid to solving the problem. Professor Cowell felt that a mere increase in income would be no solution. It would lead to the consumption of better grades of beef and more visits to the cinema.[33]

Such attitudes were, however, beginning to arouse opposition. Professor A.W. Ashby wrote to the committee protesting about the character of the discussion. To expect the poor to plan their eating by reference to strict scientific criteria and within the limits of their income was 'dogmatism on the morals of consumption'. He warned the committee that their views might be seen as justification for wage cuts. In addition,

No class in the community has ever believed that the sole purpose of eating was nutrition; none will ever do so until it is forced to do so by poverty. Even the poor, sometimes the poorest, sacrifice something of nutritive values to their tastes and social standards, and not entirely through ignorance. They choose between satisfactions, and it is not for the better-fed to say they choose wronglyh, because they would almost certainly make equally wrong choices in the same circumstances . . .

I know it is not your intention to suggest that considerations of nutrition must be the sole object of eating and I hope that it is not your intention to suggest that considerations of nutrition must dominate all others at certain levels of income. But of course many people would like to enforce the acceptance of the second principle. Fortunately the working classes have always had a realization — dim though it may be — that this is one of the principles that would carry their wages to subsistence level.[34]

Such criticisms had their effect. By 1937, at the height of the controversy about diet, PEP whilst committed to the same principles of better food distribution, special agricultural subsidies and advice as the solution to the problem of working class nutrition were willing to admit that, 'it is reasonable to suppose that a general rise in the purchasing power to persons in the lower income groups would do most to solve the problem'.[35]

What were the connections between eugenics, social hygiene and planning? According to Lindsay's history of PEP, three groups intersected at the formation of PEP. First was what Lindsay called the Blackett group; second, were those around the *Weekend Review*; and third were the group at Toynbee Hall, particularly J.J. Mallon and R.C. Davison. Of these groups,

> Sir Basil Blackett's connections were in the financial, imperial and eugenic fields (he was President of the British Social Hygiene Council). Apart from himself the only ones who worked much on PEP were Dr C.P. Blacker, Graeme Haldane and A.T.K. Grant.[36]

Blackett's eugenic connections were substantial. At a meeting of PEP on 28 January 1932 at University College, London, Blackett was in the chair and Carr-Saunders, E.J. Lidbetter, Lady Limerick, Otto May, Josiah Stamp and Mrs Neville Rolfe, all prominent eugenicists, were present. Neville Rolfe spoke with Lindsay at this meeting on 'Social Structure'. At a later meeting, 18-19 April 1932, at Dartington Hall, a study group on 'The Feebleminded' was set up consisting of Huxley, Blackett and Neville Rolfe.[37] Some of the eugenicists connected with the early years of PEP subsequently dropped out. Lidbetter, Lady Limerick, Otto May and Neville Rolfe remained members but were not deeply involved. Carr-Saunders, Blacker and Huxley were more active. By the time of Blackett's death, in a motor car accident in Germany in 1935, his links with PEP had become tenuous due partly to disagreements with Salter over the question of Imperial Preference but also to the impatience of some of the younger members with his rather conservative approach. None the less Blackett's linking of eugenics and planning continued to exercise influence in PEP.

In *Planned Money*, published in 1932, Blackett had pointed to the apparent doubling of the feebleminded since 1908 as evidence of the failure to apply rational social planning. His views were similar to those expressed by Lord Dawson of Penn (who was asked to join the NFYG but declined due to pressure of medical commitments). Dawson, during the debate on sterilisation, in 1935 complained that 'While there was a readiness to discuss planning in the sphere of economics, industry and the social services there was 'shyness' even a 'shirking' to study and determine the conditions which would produce high quality children yet unborn.'[38] Julian Huxley too made a connection between planning in the economic and the biological spheres. In a description of economic planning in 1934, which was virtually a resumé of PEP's aims, he argued that,

> Planning in the sense in which that word is generally used today is not enough. It is extremely important to plan out our cities, to rationalize our industries, to guard against exaggerated slumps and booms in the domain of finance, to make provision through cooperative marketing, production quotas, import regulations for a steady flow of agricultural products and a healthy farming industry to adjust our currency to a flexible world-system, and so on. But this alone is only one aspect of biological and social engineering. In the long run, it is equally important to plan for education, for health, for self development in adult life, for the intelligent use of the steadily increasing amount of leisure which will be available in a planned society, for quantity of population, for racial improvement.[39]

The ideas of social hygiene were closely linked to orthodox economics. Economic discussion before the First World War described unemployment as caused by the changing structure of industry, the labour market and economic depressions. But it had also frequently attributed persistent unemployment to the existence of a residuum of the morally, physically and mentally unfit. Eugenics merely gave biological expression to this idea. The most vociferous exponents of eugenics were inclined to place the whole burden of poverty and unemployment on the multiplication of the unfit. Others took a less Manichæan view of the problem of unemployment.[40] But it is true that writings on economics often included the control of the residuum by eugenic means, along with strictly economic reform, as a means to bring about economic progress.[41]

In the inter-war years the obvious structural problems of British industry, especially the impact of the economic crisis of 1931, made the problem of the residuum seem less relevant, although it did not banish it completely in either economics or in social policy. There was, however, another aspect of social hygiene which seemed perhaps more pertinent. Orthodox economics in the inter-war years emphasised the need for wage reductions to rescue Britain's industries from their uncompetitive position. After the economic crisis of 1931 it wanted government public expenditure cut to get rid of the budget deficit. Social hygiene offered a programme of reform which was sometimes tangentially but often directly related to these ideas. It attempted to teach the working class the science of reduced consumption, that it was 'possible to eat well at current wage rates'! It regarded expenditure on social welfare as needing to be scientifically assessed, that is to move away from 'largesse', as Blacker put it, to careful discrimination between individuals. It emphasised scientific breeding, living and eating, the object of which was to adjust the poor to the current economic conditions of deflation and unemployment.

Proponents of *laissez faire* had never flinched from interference, regulation and control in working class life. But it is possible that some rejected state control of fertility. This reluctance largely disappeared among exponents of advanced capitalism. The advocates of monopolisation were strongly committed to planning on all points. Moreover the rationalisation of industry would in their opinion, make control of fertility even more important. As rationalisation proceeded, two things would happen. The residuum of the unemployable would increase and these could only be got rid of by birth control and, in drastic cases, by voluntary sterilisation. In addition, the remaining work force would have to improve its efficiency to meet the demands of modern industry. This could be accomplished through health reform and better domestic management. But industrial psychology would also play a part. Leonard Darwin noted in 1912 what a potent weapon for positive eugenics industrial psychology could become.[42] In their description of the National Plan in 1931, the *Weekend Review* incorporated industrial psychology as well as eugenics as part of the rationalisation process,

> A further technical weapon required from the onset would be a strong Industrial Psychology Institute on a similar basis, to avert and eliminate mistakes in factory organization of lay-out with every facility for rapid determination of methods of reducing fatigue, increasing output and promoting welfare and health of workers and interests for their leisure time.[43]

There were various practical outcomes of the eugenics-PEP connection.

PEP had a sub group on Racial Health from 1935-6 which studied quantitative and qualitative aspects of population. Its programme of study included the differential birth rate, the possible genetic differences between social classes and mental deficiency, especially the Social Problem Group. Its eventual recommendations were the improvement of statistical data on population questions, research into the genetics of the Social Problem Group and the establishment of a racial health department at the Ministry of Health. It also wanted better distribution of birth control information, racial health teaching in schools and voluntary sterilisation of those with hereditary defects.[44] The litany of measures advocated by the Eugenics Society to bolster the middle-class birth rate was given an airing by this group — help with educational costs, more income tax rebates, child services and, with a nod at the economic and industrial sections of PEP, industrial rather than state medical insurance for fathers of families. However a degree of realism prevailed,

> Apart, therefore, from discouraging the more obvious dysgenic unions and even preventing the birth of children where the parents are mentally defective or suffer from congenital defects, it is improbable that we can expect any striking improvement in the general standard of health from eugenic measures in the near future. It is, however, important that a great deal more time and money should be devoted to the study of social biology in order that knowledge may be acquired to provide a basis for a more positive eugenic policy later on.[45]

These views were similar to the section on Genetics and Public Health which appeared in 1937 in *Britain's Health Services*, a major publication by PEP. It was moderate in tone — probably written by Huxley — but fully committed to the Brock Report whose 'genetics' it accepted. It also brought up the Social Problem Group again,

> Professor A.M. Carr Saunders and Mr D. Caradog Jones, in the revised second edition of the Social Structure of *England and Wales* (1937) accepted the findings of the Wood Committee (discussed in Chapter IX) that the incidence of mental defect in England and Wales has increased during the past generation, although it has probably not doubled. They point to the existence of a class of some hundreds of thousands, who in the words of a Board of Education Report are adding '50,000 recruits to our industrial army each year who are not only unprepared by mental retardation to meet effectually the demands of a full life, but who furnish society with the bulk of its inefficient adults, criminals, paupers, mendicants and unemployables'.[46]

Neither eugenics nor scientific eating escaped criticism in the 1930s. It was, in fact, a decade in which the precepts of social hygiene were scrutinised with an increasingly hostile eye. These criticisms were to have their effect at the end of the decade. In 1931, however, the National Government was returned with a substantial majority and proceeded to make cuts in the pay of public servants and in unemployment benefit. R.A. Fisher, although a firm supporter of the National Government, worried about the dysgenic effect which cuts in teachers' pay would have and, for a while, he wondered whether the Eugenics Society should throw its weight behind a campaign to have these restored.[47] For others the more substantial issue was the effect of cuts on the unemployed. There were about three million of these in August 1931. Thereafter the figure dropped slowly but by the mid 1930s there was still a high level of unemployment and a heavy concentration in some areas. The Government, after many squalls and back-tracks, eventually restored some of the cuts in unemployment pay but, since this was hardly generous anyway, many wondered about the effect of high unemployment on health.

A substantial battle was fought between the Government and its critics over the issue of health and unemployment in the 1930s.[48] It is still an unresolved question. Historians are still assessing what the relationship between them was. Improvement in overall health continued to show up in the statistics in the 1930s, except for several worrying years when maternal mortality rose. However, this overall picture disguised the great differences between regions and classes. In particular the differences in health between social classes widened in these years.

Special attention was focused on nutrition. In response to public clamour about the effect of the cuts on diet the Government in 1931 appointed an Advisory Committee on Nutrition. This produced in 1932 a scale of food values it considered necessary to maintain health. In 1932 the BMA appointed its own committee which published, in November 1933, its own food table plus an approximate costing. Some embarrassment ensued when the two tables were compared. Whereas the BMA suggested 3,400 calories per day and 100 grams of first class protein were needed to maintain the health of an adult male, the Ministry of Health's Committee suggested 3,000 calories and 50 grams per day. At a conference hastily convened in May 1934 to iron out these differences, the highly subjective and marginal nature of these calculations became apparent.[49] The BMA's higher figure, it emerged, had been based on the assumption that the unemployed man would expend energy on his garden allotment and in physical exercise. They had also allowed for loss of calorific value in cooking. The Ministry of Health Committee had programmed for a sedentary life. A sliding scale was then introduced by the two bodies of 3,400-4,000 calories for the active adult male to 2,600-3,000 for the inactive. The protein requirement was revised to 80-100 grams. However even these estimates differed from others available at the time. It also became clear that such tables required a close intermeshing of living and eating styles with not much margin for safety. More important was the cost per head of a diet considered nutritionally satisfactory from a calorific and protein viewpoint.

The BMA Report estimated that a man, wife and three children needed to spend £1 2s 6½d on food per week (or 4s 6d per head), excluding rent and other expenditure, to be satisfactorily fed. This figure was immediately attacked as too low. Correspondents wrote to the *BMJ* pointing out that in certain regions the diet recommended by the BMA would at current prices, cost much more. A few months before, the *Weekend Review* had produced its own costed food budget for a man, wife and two children. It had estimated an expenditure on food of 17s 6d per week (4s 4½d per head).[50] These budgets were lower than those of the People's League in 1926 but since then there had been a fall in food prices of about one-third, according to some estimates. They therefore fell within the general range envisaged by the League although, by now, some provision for tea was made, the special needs of children were accepted and there was more consciousness of vitamins.

To some observers such calculations required a superhuman effort on the part of the unemployed and low-wage earner. Or at the least it required, as Ashby said, a high degree of self abnegation. The *Weekend Review* survey, admitted as much. They worked out that it was possible for a man not engaged on heavy work to subsist on 3s 2½d a week. But to do so he would have to consume eight pints of porridge a day. As the *Weekend Review*'s investigators accepted, whilst this would satisfy calorific value it was not realistic to expect the unemployed to follow this diet.

Once the practice of fixing the cost of a nutritionally adequate diet had begun, then diets and diet sheets proliferated. The BMA followed up its investigations with a cook-book for the working-class family and the Ministry of Health sponsored a series of exhibitions on good nutritional practice. But also entering this field were organisations who were much more critical of government and official attitudes to surviving on low pay and unemployment benefit. These included the Children's Minimum Committee and the Committee against Malnutrition, which, with others, provided a stream of critical comments on official policy

in the 1930s. In particular the work of the nutritionist John Boyd Orr
and the investigations of G.C.M. McGonigle and J. Kirby on diet and
family income were frequently quoted by opponents of the Government's
policy.[51] As in the case of voluntary sterilisation, there was, for the first
time, a clear crystallisation of opinion hostile to the presumptions of social
hygiene, which produced work more publicly available and quoted than
previously. The leftward movement of opinion amongst some 1930s
intellectuals was clearly, though not exclusively, at work here.

Two very different views about the function of eating existed in the
1930s. This was revealed in the correspondence about family budgets
in the *Weekend Review* in 1933. Some letter writers were outraged by
the degree of privation in some families due to the Depression. Others
such as J.C. Pringle and Edith Corry, representatives of the Charity
Organisation Society and members of the Eugenics Society, thought that,
'benefits must be considered equitable and cannot in the present position of the national finances be increased'.[52] Edith Corry talked of the
personal faults of some of these hard cases, of the need for discrimination in helping them and the importance of family limitation as a solution.[53] Geoffrey Elton of the National Labour Party joined the debate
arguing against, 'the unreasonable agitation against the present
Government'.[54]

These beliefs persisted in the official reaction to the controversy over
nutrition. In response to public disquiet, particularly accusations of a
deterioration in the health of the depressed areas, the government
instituted a number of official inquiries. One of these put the position
of social hygiene perfectly,

> We have been impressed by the fact that such manifestations (of ill
> health) are by no means uniform but that there is a marked divergence
> between families subject to the same economic and environmental con-
> dition. A family of one household may show a high standard of health
> while that of a neighbouring household may show evidence of
> deterioration. Stress has been laid by Health Visitors and Social
> Workers on the extreme variations of household management.[55]

A reference to Cathcart's *Poverty, Nutrition and Growth* accompanied
this. The lines were drawn in a similar fashion during the debates in
Parliament on malnutrition in 1935 and 1936. Opposed to evidence of
deprivation was the insistence upon the efficiency of the household as
the determining factor in that deprivation. As Sir Kingsley Wood,
Minister of Health, said in these debates,

We often hear Sir John Orr quoted, rather incompletely, but there is another equally eminent member of the Ministry of Health Committee who can I suppose be regarded equally as an authority and that is Professor Cathcart. He says that malnutrition is due not so much to poverty as to ignorance and other causes of the same kind.[56]

By the late 1930s, however, the leftward trend among some intellectuals was having an effect. In 1938 the Eugenics Society set up a Population Policies Committee jointly with PEP. The chairman was Professor Noel Hall, now director of the National Institute of Economic and Social Research. The committee included representatives from the Eugenics Society, C.P. Blacker, Carr Saunders, now director of the London School of Economics, D.V. Glass (also a member of the Population Investigation Committee), Eva Hubback, and Caradog Jones of Liverpool University. PEP representatives included E.M.H. Lloyd of the Board of Trade, Max Nicholson and S.K. Ruck of the London County Council. The Committee was formed as a result of concern at Britain's declining birth rate.[57] The Population Investigation Committee set up in 1935 was to provide this new organisation with detailed information on the falling birth rate and differential fertility. The Population Policies Committee objective was to survey the social and economic conditions necessary to improve the reproductive power of the eugenically good in different occupational groups.

The appointment of Francois Lafitte as Secretary to the Committee in 1938 was a significant development. He was to play a similar role as devil's advocate in the Population Policies Committee to that of Hogben in the Population Investigation Committee. Lafitte was Havelock Ellis's stepson and his appointment came about as a result of the eugenic grapevine.[58] In every other respect, Lafitte was different from the usual eugenicist. He was a graduate in Politics, Philosophy and History from Worcester College, Oxford and had received a diploma in anthropology. Only twenty-four at the time of his appointment he represented the new generation of youthful radicals. Before joining the Population Policies Committee, he had worked as a researcher for trade unions and the New Fabian Research Bureau. His political sympathies were with the Labour Movement. As secretary and chief researcher for the Population Policies Committee, Lafitte had considerable influence over its direction. For example, in October 1938 he presented to the committee a document, 'Family Allowances as a Population Policy'.[59] In this he argued for allowances as a means of alleviating poverty rather than a eugenic measure except in so far, he argued, that raising the standard of living of the working classes would lead to a limitation of their families. The discussion that followed revealed a high degree of tension in the committee. Carr Saunders argued that the committee should keep to the question of the quality of the population and ignore environmental issues. Lafitte and D.V. Glass pointed out the dangers of family allowances being used to cut wages (a fear common in labour circles). Others in the committee protested that wages were being discussed in the context of family 'needs'. Wages were not determined by needs but by economic conditions. According to the Minutes, 'There was much argument about the relation between fertility and economic status.' C.P. Blacker offered to make J.A. Fraser Roberts's work on intelligence and family size available to the committee.[60]

The sniping went on in subsequent meetings. Lafitte prepared a document on the value to eugenics of improvement in working class conditions. He quoted Hogben's book on *Genetic Principles in Medicine and Social Science* and J.L. Gray's work on the pool of wasted educational ability among working class school children.[61] Carr Saunders and Blacker, in the discussion that followed, repeated their view that environment could only affect the potential not the innate capacity of the individual. Thus it was largely irrelevant to the concerns of the committee. In any case, Carr Saunders stated that the pool-of-wasted-ability theory was misconceived. Blacker said there were two groups among the working class, the respectable and the social problem group and that this should guide policy.[62] Lloyd objected to the vertical redistribution of income between social classes advocated in Lafitte's document on family allowances. He preferred horizontal redistribution, within not between, social classes from the childless to those with children. In the end the committee struck by the genius of compromise 'agreed that some sort of redistribution whether wholly vertical or wholly horizontal or both in combination seemed desirable'.[63] This suspension of the question, however empty it was, served to tide over the committee. Whilst Lafitte went back to prepare another document, the events of 1939 overtook the Population Policies Committee. It remained in existence, through meeting infrequently, during the war. By the time of its final report in 1948, the world had changed substantially.

The tension revealed by these meetings are significant for they reflect the collision between two opposed viewpoints. On the one hand was Lafitte and Glass's view of social welfare as a means of raising the consumption of the working class, of poverty as something the state or economic system had to alleviate and of the differential birth rate as a peripheral rather than central concern for social policy. On the other hand were the older generation of eugenicists and PEP stalwarts insisting on the sanctity of the existing wage system and on social hygiene as opposed to social welfare. Was there a meeting point between the two?

Richard Titmuss produced a book *Poverty and Population* in 1938 which comes nearest to reconciling the two. He combined social criticism, for example a stress on the avoidable nature of differential social class mortality and health, with eugenic 'claims'. Furthermore he both deplored the higher birth rate in the poorer depressed areas and at the same time called for more social welfare provision as a solution. At the same time what he had to say about inter-regional migration was satisfying to the most rigorous eugenicist,

> Those left behind, below the average in intelligence and physique will inter-marry and consequently tend to create clusters of the Social Problem Group. This group is the source from which all too many of our criminals, paupers, degenerates, unemployables and defectives are recruited.[64]

Huxley specialised in this kind of double-sided exegesis in the late 1930s.[65] It represents a deliberate marriage of eugenics and the more radical social philosophies of the 1930s. It was a very unstable marriage. Already in the 1940s Blacker was complaining about another book by Titmuss on similar lines though, appropriately for the 1940s, more radical in tone. He wrote in a memorandum that 'the writer makes a mistake in trying to combine a scientific treatise with a political diatribe'.[66] To Blacker, politics was what the other fellow introduced into the discussions. By then, of course, the events of the war had pushed things on even further.

Equally important in changing attitudes was the impact of Keynesianism. The publication in 1936 of Keynes's *General Theory* reopened the question of the role of government policy in times of depression. Between 1936 and the outbreak of the war in 1939 there was considerable discussion of his ideas. In 1936, the *Economist*, previously a sceptic, had conceded that,

> After the experience of the last fifteen years, it cannot be maintained that reductions in money wages alone are capable of curing unemployment. . . . The experience of recent years consequently suggests that efforts to stimulate effective demand are more likely to succeed than efforts to reduce costs.[67]

This favourable evaluation of Keynes's argument against balanced budgets and cuts in expenditure began to permeate the planning groups. Sir Alfred Salter, a figure of great importance in drawing up NFYG financial policy, publicly associated himself from 1937 with the appeals made by Keynes for government provision of public works to stave off another recession.[68] In 1933 Salter had supported public works but without any real conviction of their efficacy. In the summer of 1937 the NFYG held a conference on economic policy with the object of reconsidering their policy in the light of recent developments in economic thought. PEP also set up a Keynesian study group at that time.[69] Reconsiderations of this kind had significance for social hygiene. But they were by no means universally accepted among the planning groups. R.C. Davison, for example, was still very hostile to these ideas. In 1938, on a return from a trip to the USA he spoke slightingly of the public works policy of Roosevelt.

> The whole doctrine of work relief i.e. wage jobs created for the needy unemployed as such, is now universally challenged by thinking Americans. It can never take the place of direct relief, it encroaches on ordinary employment, public and private, its cost is terrific and it demoralizes many kinds of people, particularly the coloured man, who finds it a very comfortable way of life.[70]

Similarly, proponents of rationalisation like Molson took a highly conventional view of government monetary policy. He wrote to Clifford Allen in 1937 to argue that the government must cut back immediately on social services expenditure because of re-armament. Molson regarded inflation as the prime danger and recalled 1931 when, to avoid a budgetary crisis, he had also been in favour of a cutback in 'lavish and useless expenditure'. He did allow for a public works fund but it was of the type envisaged by the *Economist* in 1931.[71]

The NFYG, for all its dalliance with Keynesianism, ended up with a modified policy which still tried to combine financial orthodoxy with public works. In their final manifesto before the war, *Public Works and Slump Control*, they advocated two budgets, one on current expenditure balanced annually, one for 'useful' public works balanced quinquennially. The NFYG had gone some but not all of the way. A social and political crisis like the Second World War was necessary before significant change in attitude could take place.

Notes

1. C.L. Mowat, *Britain Between the Wars, 1918-1940* (University of Chicago Press Illinois, 1955), p. 433.

2. It had 52 candidates out of 515 elected on 30% of the vote. In the 1935 election it recovered some of its ground with 154 seats and 37.9% of the vote; see P. Addison, *The Road to 1945* (Cape, London, 1975).

3. See John Pinder (ed.), *Fifty Years of Economic Planning: Looking Forward, 1931-81*, and 'A History of PEP', PEP Papers, UP 10/2-10/4 for the following account.

4. Other members of the Employment Committee included H.C. Emmerson (Ministry of Labour) and Eva Hubback (Morley College, Family Allowance Movement). In 1935, L.H. Green, T.B. Martin, MP (Industrial Reorganisation League), C.S. Petherham and S.K. Ruck joined. On the Health Committee in 1934 were Dr Massey, MOH, Coventry and Dr A.L. Kerr. In 1937 they were joined by Dr R.E. Harkness, Dr Scott Williamson, Raymond Mortimer and H.T. Maling.

5. H. Molson, *National Labour Newsletter*, 27 May 1933, vol. 3 no. 5.

6. Basil Blackett, *Planned Money* (Constable and Co., London, 1932) p. 7 and 'Economic Development in Post War Britain', *Nineteenth Century and After*, vol. 118 (July-December 1935) p. 718, and pp. 734-5.

7. See H. Molson, review of 'Towards a National Policy', in *National Labour Newsletter*, 11 May 1935, vol. 7 no. 4. The five members of the National Labour Committee who drew up this document were G. Elton (NFYG) R.C. Davison, (NFYG and PEP), Alfred Zimmerman (PEP), R.D. Denman (NFYG) and K. Lindsay (PEP).

8. Allen Papers, NFYG, Allen to Barratt Brown, 31 May 1934.

9. *The Times*, 10 March 1933. The other three were Carr Saunders, Caradog Jones and Professor Hilton. Salter wrote to *The Times* on 21 March 1933 a letter favourable to the idea of public works but sceptical as to their economic benefit.

10. 'Public Works', *Economist*, vol. 112, (7 February 1931) p. 281. See 'The Government's General Task', ibid., vol. 113 (7 November 1931), p. 843 for its support of the National Government.

11. Lionel Robbins, *The Great Depression* (Macmillan, London, 1934) pp. 145-6.

12. Allen Papers, NFYG, Young to Allen, 12 December 1933, p. 3.

13. See H. Macmillan, *Winds of Change* (Macmillan, London, 1966), p. 371.

14. Allen Papers, NFYG, General Policy Committee, 21 April 1936, p. 2.

15. The Government's Economic Advisory Committee set up a committee on rationalisation, 11 August 1931. See CAB 58/175-80.

16. PEP Papers, WGIA 1932-4, Economic Division, Interim Report, 1935, 845/35 on Permissive Legislation and the Enabling Bill.

17. See H. Molson, 'Industry, Capital and Labour in the Fascist State', *English Review*, vol. 57, November 1933; and PEP Papers, UP10/2 Notes for a History of PEP: The Early Period, p. 6.

18. See *Entrance to Industry Report* and *Exit from Industry Report*, (PEP, London, May, 1935).

19. PEP Papers Civic Division, 5125/34/Social Assistance. An Outline of A Planned Employment Report, 10 December 1934.

20. H. Molson, H of C Deb, 28 February 1934, vol. 286, p. 1183.

21. *Weekend Review*, 23 August 1930, pp. 244-5.

22. Allen Papers, NFYG, General Policy Committee, 21 April 1936, p. 2.

23. See Allen Papers, ibid., 'A Programme of Priorities', 1937.

24. PEP WG 14/2-15.3. 3456/34. Social Assistance Group, 5 July 1934, p. 9.

25. Ibid.

26. Allen Papers, NFYG, General Policy Committee, 21 April 1936, p. 3.

27. Ibid., 'A Programme of Priorities', 1937.

28. PEP WG2/1, 3 December 1935, Notes on Nutrition.

29. Ibid., p. 1.

30. Ibid., F.R. Cowell 4809/34, 19 November 1934. Memo on the Need for a National Food Policy, p. 11.

31. PEP Research Group, 4798/34 Res., 17 November 1934, p. 1.

32. Ibid., p. 41.

33. *Idem*, 5046/34 Res., 7 December 1934, p. 4.

34. *Idem*, WG 2/1, Res.5368/34, 20 December 1934, Science and Food Supply, p. 1.

35. *Idem*, WG 15/5, Proposed Nutrition Policy, 28 May 1937. The nutrition controversy also had an effect on the People's League. In 1938 they set up an investigation under Dame Louise McIlroy into the effects on maternal mortality of nutritional supplements to pregnant women. The result published during the War demonstrated their value in preventing toxaemia.

36. PEP Papers UP10/2 Working Members and Contracts during the Thirties, App. 9.

37. Ibid., App. 4.

38. Address to York Medical Society, 24 October 1935.

39. Julian Huxley, 'The Applied Science of the Next Hundred Years. Biological and Social Engineering', *Life and Letters*, vol. II (October 1934), p. 45.

40. The most extreme exponent of the idea that working class poverty was the product of uncontrolled fertility was probably the Malthusian League of C.V. Drysdale, who were advocates of birth control. However by the 1920s the Malthusians, realising their unpopularity, had largely dispersed into other organisations including the Eugenics Society; see Soloway, *Birth Control and the Population Question in England*.

41. See for example Alfred Marshall, 'Thus progress may be hastened by thought and work . . . by the application of the principle of Eugenics to the replenishment of the race from its higher rather than lower strains . . .', *Principles of Economics*, 1890-5, pp. 843-4. For the influence of Darwinian biology on Marshall see G. Jones, *Social Darwinism in English Thought* (Harvester, Brighton, 1980), pp. 114, 145 and 191. For William Beveridge's ideas on the residuum and its biological control see J. Harris, *William Beveridge. A Biography* (Oxford University Press, Oxford, 1977), pp. 119-21.

42. L. Darwin, 'The Cost of Degeneracy', *Eugenics Review*, vol. 5, (1912), p. 98.

43. Supplement to the *Weekend Review*, 14 February 1931, p. ix.

44. PEP Papers, WG14/1, Population Policies and Racial Health, (CI).

45. *Idem*, WG15/2, Draft Broadsheet, 24 March 1936, p. 1.

46. *The British Health Services* (PEP, London, December 1937) p. 316.

47. Eug/C108, Blacker-Fisher Correspondence, December 1933.

48. Charles Webster, 'Healthy or Hungry Thirties?', *History Workshop*, vol. 13 (1982) pp. 110-29; J. Macnicol, *The Movement for Family Allowances, 1918-45* (Heinemann, London, 1980).

49. 'The Nutrition Question', *BMJ*, 19 May 1934, pp. 900-1.

50. *Weekend Review*, 1 April 1932, p. 358.

51. See John Boyd Orr, *Food, Health and Income* (Macmillan, London, 1936) and G.C.M. M'Gonigle and J. Kirby, *Poverty and Public Health* (Gollancz, London, 1936).

52. J.C. Pringle, *Weekend Review*, 25 February 1933, p. 198.

53. E. Corry, *Weekend Review*, 4 March 1933, p. 243.

54. G. Elton, *Weekend Review*, 24 February 1933, p. 198.

55. Report on the Investigation into the Industrial Conditions in Certain Depressed Areas, 1934 Cmnd 4728, p. 28.

56. H of C Deb, 8 July 1936, vol. 314, p. 1243.

57. The falling birth rate was the subject of considerable discussion in the 1930s; see Jane Lewis, *The Politics of Motherhood* (Croom Helm, London, 1980); Enid Charles, *The Twilight of Parenthood* (Watts and Co., London, 1934); G.F. McCleary, *The Menace of British Depopulation* (Allen and Unwin, London, 1937).

58. See Eug/C199.

59. PEP BWD 1/1-1/3 4350/38, Population Policies Committee, 9 November 1938 (Minutes of 14 November 1938).

60. Ibid., p. 3.

61. *Idem*, 4605/38, 16 November 1938 (Minutes of 28 November 1938).

62. Ibid., p. 4.

63. Ibid., p. 4.

64. R. Titmuss, *Poverty and Population* (Macmillan, London, 1938), p. 288.

65. J. Huxley, 'Eugenics and Society', *Eugenics Review*, vol. 28 (April 1936), pp. 11-31.

66. Eug/C333, note by Blacker on Titmuss, 16 November 1941.

67. 'Full Employment', *Economist*, vol. 123 (4 April 1936), p. 5.

68. *The Times*, 9 June 1937, 15 and 16 December 1937.

69. Allen Papers, NFYG, Occasional Communications No. 1, February 1938, p. 3, 'The whole question of slump prevention and slump control was the subject of an informal conference at Balliol College, last summer, held under the auspices of the 'Next Five Years Group', and it is a welcome fact that a committee of PEP is engaged upon the subject.'

70. *National Labour Newsletter*, New Series, vol. 1, no. 8, 18 June 1938, p. 198.

71. Allen Papers, NFYG, Molson to Allen, 21 June 1937.

Indeed subsidising mass consumption is much more violently opposed by these 'experts' than public investment. For here a 'moral' principle of the highest importance is at stake. The fundamentals of capitalistic ethics require that 'You shall eat your bread in sweat — unless you happen to have private means'.
(M. Kalecki, 'The Political Aspects of Full Employment', Lecture given to the Marshall Society at Cambridge 1942. Reprinted in the *Political Quarterly*, 1943, vol. 14, pp. 322-31.)

The Second World War had a profound effect on the social hygiene movement. In the first place it led to the break-up and dispersal of many of the groups. Three of the mental health organisations, the CAMW, the National Council for Mental Hygiene and the Child Guidance Clinic formed a Mental Health Emergency Committee at the outbreak of the war in 1939. Three years after, in 1942, it became the Provisional National Council for Mental Health. After the war it re-emerged as one group, dropping the 'Provisional' in its title.[1] The scope of its activities were much reduced during the war and the world it entered after 1945 was very different from that of the 1930s.

The Population Policies Committee of PEP and the Eugenics Society, was not suspended but it did not meet formally until 1942. In 1943 François Lafitte joined *The Times* — in the 1940s undergoing its radical phase under the editorship of Barrington Ward[2] — as a leader writer and thereafter could only give part-time help to the Population Policies Committee. He was replaced by Dr Jane Isaacs. During this time he was also preparing PEP's evidence to the Beveridge Committee on Social Insurance.[3] Members of the Population Committee had been dispersed in various civilian and military tasks at the outbreak of the war but by 1942 they began to drift back together. This was helped by the return of C.P. Blacker from the army in 1942. He returned to London to take up an appointment at the Ministry of Health to study the provision of mental health services in Britain. His return also signalled the revival of the Eugenics Society.[4]

The members of the People's League of Health were dispersed over various sorts of war work. Olga Nethersole spent the war with 'a travelling kitchen to teach the poorer women the value of foodstuffs'.[5] But although the People's League met to enjoy a dinner in 1942,[6] it never, as far as can be discovered, reassembled, and Olga Nethersole, its founder, died in 1951.

PEP suffered a loss of staff due to the war. Its whole-time research staff was halved and the publication of broadsheets suspended from May 1940 until February 1941. But, after some disruption, and a direct hit by a German bomb on its headquarters, it succeeded in maintaining itself intact. Of all the groups it was the one which most successfully adjusted itself to the conditions of wartime Britain. It kept its organisation in existence but, more importantly, it adjusted to the new mood sweeping Britain in the early 1940s. First, it began to broaden the circle of contacts beyond those connected with the National Government of 1931.[7] In particular, its association with the group of radical Keynesians at Cambridge — especially Thomas Balogh and Joan Robinson — began to have an effect upon the formulation of PEP's economic policy in the 1940s.

The conditions in which social hygiene found itself in the early 1940s were subversive of many of its tenets. At first, under the Chamberlain government elected in 1935 and which survived until May 1940, planning for the war had followed largely traditional lines. These are described by historians of the war economy as the belief that the war must be paid for by conventional means, that some yearly limit must be placed on expenditure and that direction of labour must be avoided at all costs.[8] Thus, in the first year or so of the war, there was still a residue of unemployment and industry was still not totally reorganised for the war effort. When the Chamberlain government fell owing to military and economic failures in 1940, this gradually changed. Churchill headed a coalition government which brought the Labour Party into the running of the war. In 1940 Bevin, head of the Transport and General Workers Union, was given the job of Minister of Labour and direction of labour was introduced. Throughout the remainder of the war unemployment virtually disappeared and a shortage of labour developed. At the same time, direction of labour, food shortages and bombing of working class areas led to an increasing emphasis on the provision of welfare facilities for the civilian population. In addition, many of the experts who had been at odds with the political ethos of the 1930s — including Keynes — were now co-opted into government.

The very considerable mobilisation for the war effort required of the British population was accompanied by the rhetoric of 'pulling together'. However, government reports on civilian morale in 1940-2 indicated radicalisation of public opinion. There was criticism of the government's handling of the war. Morale was low and there were fears about the reappearance of unemployment when the war was over. Because of this, the government decided to launch a debate on reconstruction in the post-war world. It was aimed at allaying these fears and giving positive meaning to the war effort.

'Reconstruction', like 'rationalisation' in the 1930s, became a vogue word. The government appointed a cabinet committee on post war reconstruction. From the churches to the trade unions there was discussion about it. In 1942 William Beveridge published a report on *Social Insurance and Allied Services*,[9] subsequently seen as one of the landmarks in the movement for post-war reconstruction. This report, commissioned by the government, set out proposals for a new deal in social security. It suggested a universal, state-run system of provision for sickness and unemployment, other major social welfare benefits and family allowances. Later in 1944 Beveridge published, under his own aegis, an allied document *Full Employment in a Free Society*, setting out a policy for maintaining full employment after the war.

Was there, at last, the kind of consensus emerging about progressive social change which the planners had hoped for in the 1930s? Not altogether. There was more than one plan for post-war reconstruction and a great many sections of British society firmly resisted the attractions of a full-scale social security system and government management of the economy to achieve full employment. For example the *Economist* in the 1940s noted that the reconstruction plans issuing from industry — the Executive Council of the Association of British Chambers of Commerce and the Federation of British Industries — were rationalisation dressed up in the rhetoric of post-war planning. They consisted of the staple remedies, familiar to proponents of rationalisation in the 1920s and 1930s, of amalgamation, marketing schemes and industrial self-government through a Council of Industry. The *Economist*, a free-trade journal, had always been critical of these. In its opinion they amounted to no more than the refurbishment of the old trade associations with the additional power to fix prices.[10] Planning, the *Economist* felt, must go further than this, 'Within the last few years there has been a notable confluence of opinion on the causes of cyclical depressions of trade.'[11] It went on to describe this as the belief that savings do not automatically produce investment, that under-consumption and deflation can exacerbate depression, and that government investment can stimulate private economic activity. This was the core of the Keynesian position.

But the *Economist* baulked at the full implications. It produced a plan in 1942 for public works as a counter-cyclical measure, low rates of interest and tax relief for private firms. This would keep government investment as an emergency measure and rely largely on economic incentives to private industry to boost production.[12] It looked very like the prescriptions produced by the *Economist* in 1931, and it provoked critical replies from Thomas Balogh and Joan Robinson.[13]

These two, who perhaps could be called radical Keynesians, had a considerable influence in PEP. Changes in the political climate and in their personnel brought about by the war influenced PEP's economic thought. In 1943 PEP produced a heavily Keynesian document *Employment for All*. The *Economist* wrote 'unlike the PEP publications in the past it takes up what is now the orthodox Socialist standpoint'.[14] This referred to the document's acceptance of the need for regular government spending, not merely during depressions, and of the need for a higher level of personal income for the mass of the population. This, the *Economist*, remembering its debates with the Hobsonian socialists of the 1920s, considered 'extreme sentimental economics'.[15]

These changes in PEP were significant. But they did not take place without a great deal of heart-searching. What consequences would the disappearance of unemployment have for labour discipline? Beveridge in his *Full Employment in a Free Society* (1944) considered this at some length. Full employment might lead to inflation, labour unrest and lack of discipline at work. PEP were even more preoccupied with the question. It was clear from their discussions that they felt there had to be some other ideological basis to labour discipline provided in the new society. Before the war,

> workers' irresponsibility was expressed in the widespread feeling that 'they' should pay full 'maintenance' if 'they' could not provide work, and in the behaviour of a minority who accustomed themselves to living inadequately at the public expense. On both sides these attitudes crystallized into pressure groups with vested interests and made for bad citizenship. The building of post war social security will depend on acceptance by the citizen of stronger obligations and new compulsions. If public policy *does* ensure that every citizen can enjoy the opportunities and responsibilities which can enhance his freedom by making a reality of his rights (or claims) we believe that it will be possible to bring home to the great majority of citizens appreciation of the price which must be paid.[16]

What price was to be paid? It was in fact to accept the precepts of social hygiene. According to PEP, 'their obligation to accept expert advice and skilled services, to find work, to be trained or transferred for work, to keep fit or to be speedily restored to health and independence . . . '.[17] If these precepts were followed 'there need be little cause to fear the growth of a "Santa Claus' state sapping the morale and independence of its least responsible citizens'.[18]

This is perhaps the 'old guard' speaking. However, even granted this vein of apprehension, the mood of the early 1940s pulled along with it many of those who had been defenders of thirties' austerity. R.C. Davison joined the Social Security League which was formed to fight for the implementation of Beveridge. The Social Security League also included Paul Cadbury, Hugh Molson, Edward Hutton, B. Seebohm Rowntree, Barbara Wootten, G.D.H. Cole and Ralph Wedgwood. Hugh Molson was also prominent in the Tory Reform Group which tried to retrieve the fortunes of the Conservative Party by getting it to respond favourably to the Beveridge Report.[19] Among this group of Tory reformers were some of the most vociferous defenders of the National Government's record on nutrition such as Lady Astor.[20] In response to this changing mood Kenneth Lindsay left the National Labour Party in 1943 claiming that the public were heartily sick of the epithet of National as applied to both the Party and the National Government.[21]

These were stirring times but, even then, not all who capitulated to the new mood were happy at the turn of events. Molson, for example, went to some lengths to defend the inter-war years. It was,

a period of great political and economic progress at the end of which the English working class family was better provided for than ever before. So far from this being recognised it is now the fashion to speak of the days of peace as a deplorable period when privilege and plutocracy reigned supreme and pursued a selfish and timid policy which led from unemployment to World War.[22]

Molson also argued that the blame for unemployment did not rest solely on government management of industry and world finance. He claimed that much of it rested on the refusal of men and women to be retrained and trade union restrictive practices. He also returned to the theme of discipline. Although, 'the amount of deliberate idleness before the war was not great (none the less) it will be necessary to take some steps to substitute some other discipline for that of poverty to make the idle work'.[23] Geoffrey Elton of the NFYG and National Labour Party also felt there had been a shameful undervaluation of the 1930s. He railed against the 'self-chosen planners' of the 1940s. True planning was, he felt, best expressed in the 1930s. Then there had been 'instinctive expedients designed to meet urgent problems' in contrast to the wholesale schemes of social reconstruction he considered characteristic of the war years.[24]

Several problems faced the Eugenics Society when Blacker returned to steer its fortunes in 1942. The first of these was the publication of the Beveridge Report in the same year. The proposals in the Report had obvious eugenic aspects and, in 1943, Beveridge addressed the Society. The first question that came up for discussion was family allowances — a state payment to families with children. The Eugenics Society had always favoured family allowances as a means to encourage population growth. They had campaigned in the 1920s for tax allowances or credits for children. But they insisted that family allowances should be graded according to income and occupational group so that the middle-class family with children would get proportionately more. Beveridge's proposals were for flat-rate family allowances which made no distinction between social strata and, in fact, calculated as a percentage of income, were more favourable to the poorer family. This was immediately criticised as a dysgenic measure. In reply, Beveridge expressed his willingness to consider other graded schemes on top of the flat rate one.[25]

There were other criticisms. Cecil Binney felt that the Beveridge Report was totally incompatible with eugenics because it redistributed resources away from the middle classes to the poor. Its system of benefits made no discrimination between the eugenically good or bad. Lidbetter pointed out that this could have a startling effect on the birth rate among the social problem group.[26] In opposition to these views, Titmuss and Hubback defended the Report. Hubback 'agreed that the breeding of some members of the social problem group should be restricted by sterilisation or segregation. The State medical service proposed in the Report might help in this respect', but she defended the principle of a national minimum and provision for old age, sickness and unemployment.[27]

A more immediately pressing problem for the Society (the principles of Beveridge were, except for family allowances in 1945, not put into effect until after the war) was the appointment by the government of a Royal Commission on Population in 1944. This affected, for example, the Eugenics Society's joint project on population with PEP. The Royal Commission was the outcome of fears about the decline in the British population which had been a topic of concern in the late 1930s. Blacker was anxious to steer it towards the policy of the Society. He noted, with pleasure, that, of the 15 members of the Commission, Carr Saunders, Hubert Henderson, A.W.M. Ellis and J.R. Hobhouse had close connections with either the Eugenics Society or the Population

Investigation Committee.[28] R.C.K. Ensor, also a member of the Commission, drew close to the Eugenics Society in the 1950s.[29] The eugenic connection was even stronger among the expert witnesses. They included Blacker, Eardley Holland, D.V. Glass and Kuczynski. There were also contributions from the psychologists Godfrey Thomson and Burt and from the geneticists R.A. Fisher and J.B.S. Haldane. J.A. Fraser Roberts and E.O. Lewis also gave evidence.

Carr Saunders was, however, anxious to keep some individuals away from the Commission. During the 1940s he felt increasingly disturbed at the growing distance between the political atmosphere and the Eugenics Society. He wrote to Blacker,

> My hope is that the Society will prepare a really careful exposition of the need to keep the quality problem of the population question in mind; . . . Personally I should not be inclined to make much of Lidbetter's work and I doubt whether it would be wise to distribute his book . . .[30]

Blacker wrote back critical of Lidbetter's introduction to the book but defending the book as a whole.

In fact the Eugenics Society had every reason to be satisfied with the outcome of the PEP report on population policy which appeared in 1948 and the Royal Commission which reported in 1949.[31] Whilst both included a long list of state-supported welfare schemes for mothers and children, both advocated a system of graded family allowances. In addition, the Royal Commission also included a recommendation for some form of special provision for middle-class educational expenses, although they differed on the details of this, as they did on the question of what kind of graded family allowances should be adopted. None the less both measures were based on the Commission's acceptance of the relationship between differential fertility and national intelligence. The left wing paper *Tribune* commented, 'someone palmed off on the Commission some rubbish about the comparative intelligence of different classes and they swallowed it hook, line and sinker'.[32]

The depositions on intelligence, social class and fertility were given by Godfrey Thomson, Burt, J.A. Fraser Roberts, Fisher and Haldane. They largely agreed about the higher intelligence of the better off social groups and their relative infertility. In 1944, about the time the depositions were made, the Eugenics Society and the Nuffield Foundation gave Godfrey Thomson a sum of money to conduct a survey of the intelligence of a substantial section of Scottish school children around eleven years of age. This was intended to be used as a comparison with a similar test done by Thomson in 1932 and it was presumed that it could throw light on the question of whether the mean intelligence quotient had declined over that period, as predicted by many eugenicists.[33] Carr Saunders worried about the political response to the survey if it became known that the Eugenics Society was associated with it,

> If this sort of thing could be done privately I should very greatly welcome it; but just imagine the stupid sort of thing that would probably be said if the working of the Trust were made public. In the present state of public ignorance and suspicion, I think the cause of eugenics in general might suffer.[34]

None the less the test was done and the results became available in 1947.[35]

It showed a slight increase in average IQ. Whereas 87,498 Scottish school children in 1932 had a mean IQ of 34.5, this had risen in 1947 to 36.7 for the 70,805 school children tested. Several expert witnesses returned to the Commission in 1949 to comment on this information. Haldane was the only one to recant his previous position,

> During the last five years which have elapsed since I commented on Professor Thomson's memorandum, I have devoted a good deal of work to the problem of selection. I am now in complete disagreement with his conclusions as to the effect of differential fertility.[36]

Lionel Penrose also began to reconsider his opinion on differential fertility and intelligence. In the 1930s he had accepted that a correlation existed between them but in 1947 he wrote a memorandum for a Eugenics Society symposium on the subject, doubting whether the fears about a decline in national intelligence were justified.[37] By 1955 he had begun to doubt the validity of the intelligence test itself.

> During the last fifty years the measurement of ability by tests resembling parlour games has been extremely fashionable. The most remarkable fact about tests of this sort, namely that they give unexpectedly constant results, at first led psychologists to think that they are good measurements of something fundamental called innate intelligence. This was probably quite an erroneous inference, as is now beginning to be realised. The only thing that an intelligence test measures is a person's ability on that particular test at that particular time.[38]

Thomson and J.A. Fraser Roberts, however, were not convinced that intelligence had not declined. Thomson believed that familiarity with testing accounted for the difference between the scores in 1932 and 1947. Fraser Roberts also believed that compensatory factors masked a real decline. Burt also argued this, although earlier he had denied the significance of environmental influence on test scores.[39]

More substantial problems faced the proponents of differential fertility and intelligence. On the eve of publication of the PEP report on population, W.A. Morton, a member of PEP, commented on the proposal that family allowances be graded according to income,

> With relief given as a proportion of income, the wealthier the man the greater the subsidy, the inference is that not merely does the wealthy man spend more on his children, he should be helped to do so. This seems to me an arguable proposition in the light of current egalitarian trends.[40]

These egalitarian trends were to perplex the Eugenics Society in the years that followed.

In 1952, Blacker reported to the Eugenics Society how, in 1947, he was sent some documents by Lord Moran who had been appointed to a committee to consider Nazi war crimes.[41] These documents related to eugenic experiments and practices in Germany and Moran wanted Blacker's opinion on their scientific value. The documents Blacker received were about German sterilisation under the 1933 law, and experiments on living subjects, which took place in the 1940s, to find a cheap and quick method of sterilisation. Blacker was deeply upset at the revelations contained in these documents and wrote back to say that the experiments described in them had no scientific value. None the less he felt eugenics would suffer from its association in the public mind with the Nazi experiments. In 1939, however, he had written to Carr Saunders, 'I think it would be a good thing if the impression were removed that as a Committee we disparage the results of the German policy. For my part I regard these as substantial and indeed remarkable.'[42]

What then had gone wrong? First the Eugenics Society had never advocated compulsory sterilisation nor — in spite of one or two voices raised in favour — the lethal chamber for the insane, mental deficient or those crippled by an hereditary physical disability.[43] Nor did they share the racial bias of the Nazi. In addition, they retained a belief in ethical limits to the medical regime which ruled out experimentation on live subjects as part of normal medical practice. So far, Blacker had every reason to believe that British eugenics should be exonerated from association with Naziism.

None the less, the evidence of these documents showed that the majority of these German incidents began at the start of the war and grew as the war progressed, stimulated by an atmosphere of increasing political paranoia. It was also pushed along by the political enthusiasms of some medical men. Had there not been in British eugenics a similar emotional overstatement and a dogmatic insistence on the relationship between the survival of civilisation and the elimination of the unfit? Did not eugenics give a similar latitude to the medical man and were not some of these prepared to go further than official eugenic policy? Some eugenicists at the outbreak of the war had lamented the death of the eugenically best on the battlefield and talked of the need to retrieve the loss somehow. What would have happened if, under a different political regime, cracks in the social fabric brought about by the war had appeared? Penrose in *Mental Defect* had thought there was a strong psychological component to the demand for sterilisation of the mentally deficient and some of the descriptions members of the Society gave of the feebleminded show considerable evidence of personal revulsion, distaste and even hatred.[44] It was not possible to imagine a replication in Britain of Nazi policy towards Jews but it was possible to imagine similar treatment towards the mentally deficient.

Moreover the political character of eugenics had become more exposed. In the 1920s it was possible to include within the term 'progressive' prophets of advanced capitalism, proponents of the application of science to human affairs, the advocates of frankness about sexuality, and those favourable to state intervention, all of whom were well represented in the eugenics movement. The 1930s had sharpened the distinctions within these categories between those who believed in economic equality and major social reconstruction and those who did not. By the 1940s the apparent commitment of the Coalition war-time government to full employment, the advance of trade union rights, social welfare and greater equality brought to the fore, far more starkly than previously, the fact that eugenics put different values on social groups, regarded social problems as intractable because of their hereditary nature and advocated a very narrow and partisan approach to social reform.

The election of a Labour government in 1945 put a seal on some of the changes promised during the debate on reconstruction in the early 1940s. Blacker found it difficult to relaunch the policy of the Eugenics Society in these changed conditions. In his semi-official report on the

British mental health services published in 1947, *Neurosis and the Mental Health Services*, Blacker, besides recommending the expansion of mental hygiene, inserted into the report the recommendations of the Wood Report on the social problem group. In 1947, the Society set up a Problem Families Committee to investigate families who exhibited 'intractable ineducability', instability of character and multiple social problems.[45] Five studies in various regions were undertaken. The project was essentially a revival of the Wood Report but brought up to date by references to the problems encountered among families evacuated from the cities to the country during the war. The name was also changed to 'families' as opposed to 'social group' and this reflected Blacker's observation in 1949 that whereas the public were reluctant to make social deductions from such studies, they could be interested in individual problems, particularly child neglect.[46] However he found that some of his researchers were shy of deducing hereditarian explanations from their data. Blacker wrote to the Bristol Medical Officer of Health who conducted one of the surveys.

Are we really as ignorant as you say about the causes of the 'problem families'. If, in fact, these families exhibit the qualities of intellectual subnormality, instability of character and intractable educability, can we not say that these are in fact causative? . . . The triad of characteristics which were mentioned as our criteria in the selection of these families could be expected to appear in a small proportion of families inhabiting any industrial community so far as innate qualities are in a biological sense variable. I much doubt whether sociological researches, however well conceived and competently carried out, could throw much more light on the position.[47]

These studies were completed by 1951. However E.O. Lewis advised against publication because, 'it is as well to bear in mind that the subject of problem families and its cognate the Social Problem Group, is becoming a favourite "Aunt Sally" with a certain group of scientists of a certain political hue'.[48] Blacker, commenting sourly on these reservations in the margin of the letter, claimed 'Lewis seems (or has shown himself to be) unduly scared of these'.[49] None the less, Blacker faced a similar blockage in his attempts to revive the issue of sterilisation. In 1952 he organised a symposium to discuss the implementation of the Brock Report. He wrote to various individuals about the issue. In 1956, however, he admitted defeat. In a memorandum written jointly with Cecil Binney he stated,

Three years ago, one of us made tentative enquiries of some of the people who, from 1934-39, had served on the Joint Committee on Voluntary Sterilisation as to whether they thought the time had come to revive the committee. All responded with an emphatic negative.[50]

The leaders of the Eugenic Society occasionally pondered the significance of these changes in the political atmosphere. The icons of the new social order were, after all, Beveridge and Keynes, both of whom had taken an interest in eugenics at various stages in their careers. Keynes, in particular, had remained a member of the Eugenics Society until his death and had helped the Society with its financial affairs. The relationship between Keynes and eugenics was discussed by Blacker and Carr Saunders shortly after Keynes's death in April 1946. It puzzled them that this representative of welfarism and full employment had remained a member. Carr Saunders made a number of suggestions about the reasons. The Darwins and the Keyneses were both Cambridge families. Presumably this meant a vestigial loyalty on Keynes's part to Leonard Darwin, the first president of the Eugenics Society. Keynes was a statistician and admired Galton. He was worried about over-population. But the main reason, according to Carr Saunders was, 'He probably thought that the Society was concerned with the attempt to bring science into human affairs and that was good enough for him.'[51]

However, Carr Saunders failed to give due regard to Keynes's views. He was not a radical Keynesian in the sense in which Kalecki, Balogh and Joan Robinson were and therefore probably believed in the value of population control as a weapon of economic policy, even if full employment made it increasingly irrelevant. Beveridge's views, however, had changed substantially in the late 1930s. But although he had moved significantly leftwards, Beatrice Webb perhaps exaggerated when she wrote in her diary in 1940, 'Beveridge is today a Socialist. He agrees that there must be a revolution in the economic structure of society.'[52]

A great deal of the impasse in which eugenics found itself in the 1950s was due to changes in mental deficiency policy. Between 1945 and 1953 there was a shortage of accommodation and staff in mental deficiency institutions. This had begun in 1939 when, at the outbreak of the war, resources were diverted to deal with other more pressing problems. In response to this the number of discharges rose as did those on licence outside the institution. These administrative problems did not go away after the war. Ascertainment and notifications increased but existing accommodation did not expand. In a House of Commons Debate of 19

February 1954, the waiting list for places in mental deficiency institutions was said to be 9,000.[53]

These problems, including dissatisfaction of families who could not get a place for a relative or child in an institution, were catalysts for major changes in mental deficiency policy. In 1954 a Royal Commission on the Laws Relating to Mental Illness and Mental Deficiency was set up. This reported in 1957, when it recommended a relaxation in the policy of institutionalisation and a greater emphasis on voluntary admission. In 1959 a Mental Health Act embodied some of these proposals.

But these were by no means the only force for changes in the 1913 Act. In 1913, and in 1927, opposition to mental deficiency policy was led by Josiah Wedgwood. In the 1930s there were rumblings of discontent expressed in Parliament from time to time. In 1938, for example, a married man aged 31, William Hargraves, was arrested in a Liverpool labour exchange and returned to a mental deficiency institution. He had been certified in 1925 at age 18, released on licence from 1926 to 1934 and in that year had absconded because his licence was revoked. His case was raised in Parliament and he was eventually released.[54]

In the 1940s parliamentary questions hostile to the 1913 Act intensified. These were not just about shortage of places but raised wider issues including unjustified certification, removal of parental rights and exploitation of the labour of high-grade patients in mental deficiency institutions and outside, on licence. Part of the reason was a clear change in public perception of the possibilities open to high-grade mental defectives and this was almost entirely due to the fall in unemployment brought about by the War. In Britain unemployment in 1939 had been 11.7 per cent. In 1941 it fell to 2.2 per cent, and by 1944 it was 0.5 per cent. In 1955, it was still only 1.1 per cent. In these circumstances, the apparently ineducable and unemployable were rapidly absorbed into the labour market, a fact noticed by some mental deficiency authorities. The prediction made by J.B.S. Haldane that the cure of unemployment would alter perceptions of 'social incapacity' was borne out by these events. A deputy MOH for the County of Gloucester, J.S. Cookson, writing in 1945 claimed that, 'as a result of shortage of man power some of those who before the war could have been looked on as unemployable are now in full work'.[55] The author of this article listed the jobs obtained by certified mental deficients. They included, to Cookson's surprise, errand boy, tractor driver and warehouse checkman as well as the usual run of factory jobs. In one case, the certified mental deficient was earning more than the welfare worker assigned to visit him. This description was accompanied by a criticism of the 21st Annual Report of the

CAMW in 1934 which said it was only possible for mental deficients to work if supervised by trained workers. On the contrary, 'it is rather that in the normal peacetime labour market they are unable to get the jobs for which they are suited'.[56] Some medical practitioners complained that, now the patient was a potential economic asset, their families were reluctant to see them disappear into a mental deficiency institution. True, the individual could be put to work inside the institution or outside on licence to an employer. However, wages were not competitive in mental deficiency hospitals and often the same was true in work picked out by the institution for the patient and done outside on licence. This was probably the origin of frequent accusations that the mental deficiency authorities exploited the cheap labour of the patients.[57] Just how different wages and conditions were can be illustrated in the evidence given by the National Council for Civil Liberties in their evidence to the Royal Commission. They cited the case of

> Beatrice, sent to a hostel on licence and employed as a non-residential domestic servant at £1 5s per week, 12s 6d of which paid to the hostel. After running away got a job at £6 per week. Picked up by police and returned to the institution and no doubt credited with social inefficiency for having changed her job.[58]

Similarly, there was the case of Betty who, the NCCL alleged, had her licence revoked because she joined a trade union. This was hotly disputed by some Commission members but not the fact of Betty's wages. On the subject of Betty, the NCCL quoted the report made on her to the Board of Control.

> a male employee . . . persuaded Betty and three other domestics to join the National Union of Domestic Workers. This had disastrous results as far as Betty was concerned. She does not appear to understand her action beyond knowing she must pay her 4d per week and the regulations for work etc. demanded by the Union make it quite impossible for her (the employer) to keep or to exercise adequate supervision. She must now be paid nearly £5 per week and after paying for her board and lodging etc. this means she has £2 18s per week to spend. She must now work 8 hours in a continuous stretch. This means she had every morning or afternoon off on alternate weeks, plus one whole day a week off duty. As she (the employer) reasonably points out, she cannot supervise the patient adequately during the long off duty periods and her interest in the opposite sex (NB the woman

is 46 years old) coupled with a considerable amount of spending money, makes this desirable.[59]

In their evidence to the Royal Commission, the NCCL stated that their interest in mental deficiency began in 1947 as the result of correspondence with a hospital chaplain and the London Legal Advice Centre. Press publicity followed and requests for help increased.[60] In June 1950 they held a conference which led to the publication of the pamphlet *50,000 Outside the Law* in 1951. This detailed 400 cases of disquiet at certification but also a greater number, 3,527, urgently requiring places in an institution of whom two-thirds were, they claimed, low-grade patients. The publicity resulting from the NCCL's efforts led to complaints from some of the medical profession.

The *BMJ*, discussing the NCCL's pamphlets, objected that 'since the war the rate of discharge has been greatly accelerated and in addition all know that the Acts were due for an overhaul'.[61] But some medical men believed that mental deficiency policy ought to be criticised. L.T. Hilliard, physician superintendent of the Fountain Hospital, stated in 1954, that,

A scrutiny of the medical certificates which originally formed the basis for the detention of these patients makes one wonder if enough care was given in some cases to the evidence on which diagnosis of mental defect was based. . . . Mental deficiency practice has consolidated within the framework and experience of an Act designed 40 years ago in very different social circumstances. This has resulted in a wastage of human capabilities which I believe can in more favourable circumstances, be developed and utilised to better advantage both to the individual and the community. Mental deficiency of the so-called feeble minded category is in many cases not a clear cut clinical entity of an irreversible nature. Too often, as I have tried to show, it is the diagnosis which has created the disease.[62]

The difficulties of correct diagnosis were again raised by the findings of a MRC investigation by Tizard and O'Connor. They had used IQ tests on 12,000 patients in mental deficiency institutions. Of the 12,000, 58 per cent were high-grade and of these about half had an IQ of above 70 and, therefore, fell within the range of IQ scores found in a normal population.[63]

There was a clear perception among professional bodies that attitudes had changed. In their memorandum to the Royal Commission, the

National Association for Mental Health stated that reform was overdue because of three factors of which one was 'the state of public opinion on the extent to which interference with the liberty of the subject is necessary'.[64] Lord Eustace Percy, the chairman of the Commission conceded that the term ' ''social inefficiency'' is usually a term of political heresy'.[65]

Other factors intervened. In 1948 the Mental Health Services were reorganised under the National Health Service. This reduced the influence of some of the structures associated with the old system. The CAMW now reorganised under the Mental Health Association lost many of the functions designated to it under the 1913 Act. It turned to education, training courses and propaganda. The Mental Hospitals Association disappeared too, to be replaced by Hospital Management Committees, appointees of Regional Hospital Boards. Similarly there was a growth in salaried social workers — the mental health worker was to receive many of the powers, under the new Mental Health Act of 1959, previously exercised by the old Mental Deficiency Committees. In other words there was an attenuation of the old, middle-class, amateur, charitable organisations which, in some cases, had been semi-official arms of the State. This and the broader political representation in local government after 1945 was a factor for change.

The Royal Commission on Mental Health did not sweep away the presumptions of social hygiene but it changed them substantially. First, there was general agreement that idiots and imbeciles needed some form of supervision or help. This group was rechristened the severely subnormal. But what of the feebleminded? The NCCL recommended that the category be abolished altogether. They believed that only severely impaired intelligence should be the subject of a new Mental Health Act and that the normal process of law should take care of any other cases.

The Commission rejected this. What they did was to introduce 'behaviour disorder' or what they called psychopathy as a major new definition. This was to cover all cases previously covered by the term 'moral defective' or 'moral imbecile' and also some definitions of feeblemindedness by reason of social inadequacy. They fully admitted that this threw intelligence largely out of the window.

Feebleminded patients, moral defectives or psychopaths may be described medically as patients suffering from emotional immaturity or instability; their emotions are warped or blurred, over inhibited or over controlled. This emotional disorder may be combined with some limitation of intelligence or with some specific form of mental illness.[66]

This definition had some connection with the original 1913 category of social inadequacy but it was much more a definition of emotional and psychological disturbance than of social inadequacy by reason of low intelligence. The truly feebleminded became less central to the conception of 'mentally deficient'. According to one witness 'all high grade defectives are psychopaths'.[67] To another, the condition manifested itself because of a social environment which failed to cater for normal emotional growth.[68]

Mental hygiene began to replace social hygiene. Those of low intelligence were no longer a major social threat. Most of society had a chance to achieve full citizenship. Yet, on the way, incorrect child rearing, emotional and physical neglect, bad impressions or influences deflected the individual from the correct path of development. This meant there was much more emphasis upon individual therapeutic treatment. It also led to two other pervasive themes of the 1950s, the ideal of the normal family with the accompanying controversy over the effect of working mothers on children. The second was the preoccupation with the effect of mass culture, especially television, on the young.

In addition to these problems, the Eugenics Society secretary was losing the battle to keep at least cordial relations with Penrose. Penrose in 1945 became Galton Professor of Eugenics at University College, London much to the satisfaction of J.B.S. Haldane who had strongly supported his candidature.[69] Blacker hoped to keep on good terms with Penrose but differences arose between them over eugenics. Penrose wrote to Blacker in 1946 that 'my own experience is that eugenic prognosis is much more often a guess about the social value of the offspring rather than mathematical calculation of the chances of Mendelian inheritance'.[70] Blacker wrote back, 'as I understand your outlook as expressed at the Galton Lecture, you would largely dissociate yourself from the view that eugenics should be a factor in either social policy or religion'.[71]

The difference in their views looked like an insuperable obstacle to cooperation between Penrose and the Secretary of the Eugenics Society. None the less Blacker kept some lines open to Penrose. He offered him the opportunity to lecture to the Society whilst advising him to keep to subjects of a strictly scientific nature. By 1950, however, relations had deteriorated even further. Penrose in that year published an article on mental deficiency in the September 30 issue of the *Lancet* criticising the idea of the social problem group and the decline in national intelligence. In that year Blacker wrote to Tredgold,

> The attitude adopted by Penrose is indeed a problem. One does not wish to revive the acrimonious polemics between the Laboratory and Society which went on in the early days of both organisations. At the same time, one does not wish the impression to get around that there is no answer to the contention which Penrose advances. Holding the views he does he really had no business to accept Galton's chair.[72]

Blacker took some comfort from the difficulties J.B.S. Haldane got into in 1948 over the Lysenko affair. Editorials about the pernicious influence of left wing and environmentalist views in biology appeared in the *Eugenics Review*. In addition, Blacker, through the influence of his friend John R. Baker, became involved in the right wing Society for Freedom in Science, an organisation dedicated to reducing left wing influence in science.[73] Many of his colleagues received a letter commending John Baker's work for this organisation and Blacker himself became a financial contributor to the Society for Freedom in Science.

Blacker was also keen to salvage the reputation of eugenics for posterity. Both he and Carr Saunders were anxious in case the Home University Press's reissue of a revised volume on eugenics would be written by its opponents. Carr Saunders was fearful that 'the editors may put the revision or the rewriting of the book into the hands of someone like Haldane or Hogben which would have disastrous results'.[74] Blacker wrote his book, *Galton, Eugenics and After* published in 1952 with this current controversy very much in mind. He wrote to Carr Saunders 'I was provoked to write a refutation of the apparent misrepresentation which I believe to be partly deliberate of Galton's views on the subject by some of the communists in Penrose's laboratory.'[75] Later, he went on 'You will see that I have considered at some length the criticism of environmentalists and Hogben-minded people'.[76]

Gradually the Eugenics Society began the process of re-adjustment. Its rhetoric shifted. It became less concerned with the solution of large-scale social problems and more with the prevention of individual misfortune. Blacker had an intuition of the need for this kind of change when he wrote in 1949:

> If mothers of problem families are physically worn out by household duties to which they are unequal, and if a series of unwanted children

has contributed to reducing their physical health to a low level, could they not be sterilised on voluntary or therapeutic (not eugenic) grounds.[77]

A new generation of eugenicists was to advocate the control of reproduction in this light, as an extension of individual freedom rather than as part of an overall social strategy for improving the race. By the 1950s the ideology of the Eugenics Society had shifted significantly in this direction leaving the 'old guard' in an isolated position.

Even the influx of black and Asian immigrants into Britain in the 1950s produced only minor perturbations. Bishop Barnes of Birmingham became very agitated about it and addressed the Society on the subject of racial decay. But he was severely criticised for his views.[78] The issue of immigration and the Eugenics Society's lack of action on it brought John Baker close to resignation. He wrote to the secretary, then C.G. Bertram, in the late 1950s complaining about the censorship of his letters to the *Eugenics Review*, 'I consider that the Society has become too diffident about putting forward a bold eugenic policy, and has bowed too much to modern eugenic propaganda about the equality of all men of all races.'[79] Baker conducted a controversy for several years over the direction the Eugenics Society was taking. In 1961 he wrote again to Bertram to ask 'Do the important people in the Society really think that the political outlook of the times with its stress on egalitarianism makes direct eugenic propaganda hopeless?'[80] The answer to this question was, on the whole, yes.

A generation was gradually bowing out. Olga Nethersole died in 1951. Her memorial service was attended by Dame Louise MacIlroy, Mrs Neville Chamberlain, Lady Fripp and Lady Arthur Robinson.[81] In the same year Evelyn Fox retired from the Mental Health Association. Mrs Hume Pinsent's daughter Lady Adrian served on the Royal Commission on Mental Illness and Mental Deficiency in 1954 as did Lord Eustace Percy, both of whom proved sensitive to the criticisms of the NCCL about the operation of the 1913 Act. But the older generation of mental and social hygienists were disappearing. Mrs Neville Rolfe's Social Hygiene Council disbanded in 1950 to become the Social Biology Council. The mixture of social purity and racial progress which characterised it could not survive the 1940s, and in the war the government gave precedence to the Central Council for Health Education as the means for combating VD. Some organisations adapted and survived. The NIIP's work became more, not less, significant in an era of full employment. PEP also survived. Its collection of data and intelligence expanded during and after the war. In addition it provided a powerful prototype of an intelligence assessment unit, one frequently copied in the post-war years.

The classic theorist of the changes which took place in social policy in the 1940s was T.H. Marshall. Marshall argued in *Citizenship and Social Class*, published in 1950, that the reforms of the 1940s were the culmination of a long process which began with the extension of political rights to all, rich and poor alike.[82] This was complemented by the extension of economic rights to all, expressed in the state's commitment to providing social welfare and guaranteeing a minimum of economic security. Whilst this did not involve economic equality, the end of class differences or of the capitalist system, it had led to the mitigation of harsh economic policies, a diminution of gross inequality and to a new political stability based on the idea of a common citizenship. This was perhaps the most optimistic view of the achievements of the 1940s and the implications of them for the future.

But the consensus emerging out of the 1940s was unstable. Marshall pointed out that the working classes would have to accept duties in return for the advantages they received under this system. For example, they should eschew industrial militancy. Moreover in the same year, 1949, as he set out his views on citizenship in the Alfred Marshall lectures which were published later as *Citizenship and Social Class*, Marshall was also arguing that any more public expenditure would lead to economic stagnation. The burden of welfare should consequently be shifted back onto voluntary charitable provision.[83] In 1945 Marshall had also joined the Eugenics Society, strangely enough at the moment of its lowest social influence.[84]

There was, in fact, an undercurrent of dissatisfaction at the welfare state revealed particularly in criticisms of its cultural effects in the 1950s.[85] None the less, whilst full employment lasted and commitment to the welfare state was an important part of the programmes of all political parties, the precepts of social hygiene seemed to have been superseded. But what would happen when deflation, unemployment and stricter government budgeting reappeared?

Notes

1. Kathleen Jones, *A History of the Mental Health Services* (Routledge and Kegan Paul, London, 1972), pp. 267-8.
2. The role of *The Times* in the Second World War is discussed in Angus Calder,

The People's War (Cape, London, 1969), pp. 337-8.

3. See PEP Papers, Bulletin No. 125, The War Time Record and After, January-February 1947.

4. See *Eugenics Review*, Notes of the Quarter, vol. 35 (April 1943).

5. *The Times*, 11 January 1952.

6. Ibid., 16 December 1942.

7. See PEP Papers, *Membership and Contacts List 1939-45*. New contacts included J.D. Bernal, E.H. Carr, Lord Keynes, Professor R.A. Tawney and Sir John Boyd Orr. All were critics of the government's pre-war record.

8. W.K. Hancock and M.M. Gowing, *The British War Economy* (Longmans Green and Co. and HMSO, London, 1949); see also Paul Addison, *The Road to 1945* (Cape, London, 1975) and Angus Calder, *The People's War, Britain 1939-45* (Cape, London, 1969).

9. José Harris, *William Beveridge, A Biography* (Oxford University Press, Oxford, 1977).

10. *Economist*, vol. 142 (6 June 1942).

11. Ibid., vol. 143 (3 October 1942), p. 408.

12. 'Full Employment, the Means', *Economist*, vol. 143 (10 October 1942), p. 438.

13. *Idem*, vol. 143 (28 November 1942), pp. 662, 664.

14. *Idem*, vol. 145 (10 July 1943), p. 36.

15. Ibid., p. 69. J.A. Hobson, a Liberal, argued that British capital sought investment overseas because of low consumption at home. Raise the consumption at home by high wages, low unemployment and social reform, then the problems of Imperialism and of poverty would both be solved. Hobson had considerable influence over the economic thought of the left wing Independent Labour Party in the 1920s.

16. *Planning*, Broadsheet no. 190 (1942).

17. Ibid., pp. 9-10.

18. Ibid., p. 10.

19. See H. Kopsch, *The Approach of the Conservative Party to Social Policy during World War Two*, Unpublished PhD thesis, University of London, 1970.

20. Astor consistently depreciated the contribution of poverty to malnutrition. See H of C Deb, 17 July 1935, vol. 304, p. 1131. She was a supporter of sterilisation as was D. Gunston, another Tory reformer. See H of C Deb, 13 April 1937, vol. 322, pp. 838-40.

21. Kenneth Lindsay, 'Why it Happened', *Spectator*, 3 August 1945, p. 101. 'No party will ever again arrogate to itself the title "National" . . . The people are heartily sick of the pretence.'

22. 'Years of Progress', *The Nineteenth Century and After*, vol. 133 (April 1943), p. 161.

23. 'The Beveridge Plan', *The Nineteenth Century and After*, vol. 133 (January 1943), pp. 28-9.

24. Lord Elton, 'Reflections on a New Social Order', *Fortnightly Review*, vol. I, (May 1941), p. 457. 'The unflattering suggestion that we shall only fight whole heartedly if we are guaranteed a series of highly controversial post war changes which will put an end to Britain as we know it, usually carries with it the curious suggestion that the old Britain to which we said goodbye in September 1939, was a shameful example of social inertia and backwardness.'

25. Sir William Beveridge, 'Eugenic Aspects of Children's Allowances', *Eugenics Review*, vol. 34 (16 February 1943), p. 117.

26. 'The Eugenics Aspects of Social Security. A Discussion of the Beveridge Report', *Eugenics Review*, vol. 36 (18 January 1944), pp. 17-23.

27. Ibid., p. 23.

28. *Eugenics Review*, vol. 36 (April 1944), p. 3.

29. See R.C.K. Ensor, 'Some Problems of Quantity and Quality in the British Population', *Eugenics Review*, vol. 42 (1950), p. 125.

30. Eug/C57, Carr Saunders to Blacker, 16 June 1944.

31. See 'Population Policy', *Planning*, Broadsheet No. 281 (1948) and Report of the Royal Commission on Population, Cmnd 7695, 1949.

32. *Tribune*, 24 June 1949, quoted in *Eugenics Review*, vol. 41, no. 3 (October 1949).

33. *The Trend of Scottish Intelligence*, A Comparison of the 1947, 1932 surveys of the Intelligence of Eleven Year Old Pupils (results available in 1947) (University of London Press, London, 1949).

34. Eug/C57, Carr Saunders to Blacker, 25 June 1947.

35. Papers of the Royal Commission on Population, Cmnd 7695, 1949, vol. V, (1950).

36. Ibid., p. 43.

37. See Eug/C271.

38. *Heredity and Environment in Human Affairs*, The Convocation Lecture, (National Children's Home, London 1955), p. 18.

39. Papers of the Royal Commission on Population, Memoranda of May 1945. Burt predicted a decline of 0.87 over 20 years. As regards those who believed environment affected results they 'might argue with some plausibility that the apparent amount of decline must form an underestimate' (p. 63).

40. PEP Papers, PW 51/4, 2339/40, 19 April 1947.

41. Blacker, 'Eugenic Experiments conducted by the Nazis on Human Subjects', *Eugenics Review*, vol. 44 (April 1952), pp. 9-19.

42. Eug/C58, Blacker to Carr Saunders, 8 February 1939.

43. The exception was R.J.A. Berry, who was rapped over the knuckles by the Eugenics Society, *Eugenics Review*, vol. 22 (1930), p. 6, for his advocacy of it. Tredgold in his textbook *Mental Deficiency* discusses the lethal chamber briefly but makes no recommendations one way or another.

44. 'If it was said that sterilisation was an affront to the dignity of humanity, we should listen and agree . . . But what dignity have the feeble in mind that legislation can deprive them of it? . . . An intelligent and healthy dog is more spiritually akin to man, has more natural dignity than one of these. It is the existence of the feebleminded which affronts human dignity'. 'Notes of the Quarter', *Eugenics Review*, vol. 20 (April 1928), p. 76.

45. Eug/D169, Problem Families, Committee set up November 1947.

46. Eug/D171, 23 December 1949.

47. Ibid., Blacker to the Deputy MOH, Bristol, 23 December 1949.

48. Ibid., Lewis to Blacker, 1 February 1952.

49. Ibid., Marginalia in letter.

50. Eug/C22, Memorandum, 27 June 1956.

51. Eug/C57, Carr Saunders to Blacker, 16 May 1946.

52. Quoted in José Harris, *William Beveridge, A Biography*, p. 366.

53. H of C Deb, 19 February 1954, vol. 523, p. 2301.

54. See the *Lancet*, 2 April 1938, p. 811 and H of C Deb, 14 March and 1 April 1938, vol. 333, pp. 1627-8.

55. J.S. Cookson, 'Supervision of Mental Defectives in the Community', *BMJ*, 20 January 1945, p. 91.

56. Ibid.

57. See H of C Deb, 28 January 1957, vol. 563, p. 651.

58. Royal Commission on the Laws relating to Mental Illness and Mental Deficiency 1954, Cmnd 169, Minutes of Evidence, p. 829.

59. Ibid., pp. 809-10.

60. See Royal Commission on Mental Illness and Mental Deficiency, Minutes of Evidence, p. 793. For the publicity see *The Times*, 21 September 1953.

61. This point is discussed in the *BMJ*, 21 April 1951, p. 872.

62. L.T. Hilliard, 'Resettling Mental Defectives. Psychological and Social Aspects', *BMJ* , 12 June 1954, p. 1374.

63. N. O'Connor and J. Tizard, 'A Survey of Patients in Twelve Mental Deficiency

Institutions', *BMJ*, 2 January 1954, p. 16.

64. Royal Commission on Mental Illness and Mental Deficiency, Minutes of Evidence, p. 466.

65. Ibid., para 2446, p. 48.

66. Royal Commission on Mental Illness and Mental Deficiency, Report, para 167, p. 52.

67. Ibid., p. 53.

68. Ibid.

69. See Penrose Papers 136, Correspondence with Haldane.

70. Eug/C271, Penrose to Blacker, 25 January 1946.

71. Ibid., Blacker to Penrose, 28 January 1946.

72. Eug/C338, Blacker to Tredgold, 13 October 1950.

73. See *Eugenics Review*, vol. 40, no. 4 (January 1949), pp. 175-8; see also Eug/C13, Baker to Blacker, 26 June 1946. For an account of this controversy, see G. Jones, 'British Scientists, Lysenko and the Cold War', *Economy and Society*, vol. 8, no. 1 (1979), pp. 26-58.

74. Eug/C57, Carr Saunders to Blacker, 3 August 1943.

75. Ibid., Blacker to Carr Saunders, 25 November 1949.

76. Ibid., Blacker to Carr Saunders, 7 December 1949.

77. Eug/D171, 23 December 1949.

78. See 'The Mixing of Races and Social Decay', *Eugenics Review*, vol. 41, no. 1 (April 1949).

79. Eug/C10, Baker to Bertram, 14 August 1960.

80. Ibid., 1 February 1961.

81. *The Times*, 11 January 1951.

82. Alfred Marshall, *Citizenship and Social Class* (Cambridge University Press, Cambridge, 1950).

83. A. Marshall, 'Voluntary Action', *Political Quarterly*, vol. 20 (1949), p. 33.

84. See Eug/C227.

85. See for example N.A. Smith, 'Theory and Practice of the Welfare State', *Political Quarterly*, vol. 22 (1951), p. 376.

8 CONCLUSION

This book has attempted to answer the question of what happened to social Darwinism. Did the period of European history from the late-nineteenth century until the early-twentieth during which the concepts of heredity, Darwinian evolution and struggle for existence were popular, leave any legacy in the policies and institutions of nations? In Britain's case it is clear that it did. Social Darwinism entered the language of legislators, churchmen, politicians, medical men, charity workers, policy formers and opinion makers. Whilst social Darwinian ideas were never the only guide to the formation of medical and social policy, nor even necessarily the major guide, they were influential.

There were, of course, many social philosophies which claimed Darwinian ancestry. It is necessary to distinguish between them and, in particular, to evaluate their different social impacts. That is why social hygiene is a better name for the practical social Darwinism of our health reformers. Their ideas arose from a marriage between the social Darwinism which stressed heredity, fitness and racial progress and the practical techniques of social management which evolved from the nineteenth-century tradition of public health and charity work. It represents a blend of these two traditions.

The influence of social hygiene was possible precisely because it was easily integrated into the discourse of nineteenth-century health reform. The public health reformer of the nineteenth century urged the poor to be thrifty, far-seeing, hard working as well as physically and mentally healthy. At the same time, the public health reformer discovered the residuum. The residuum were those among the working class whom no admonition, advice, discipline or instruction seemed able to save from unemployment, immorality and ill health. These concepts easily dovetailed with the type of social Darwinism which divided the nation into the fit and the unfit and which, although it believed some of the unfit could presently be made fitter, attributed the existence of the residuum largely to heredity. This social Darwinism offered a new jargon, and scientific underpinning to the nineteenth-century tradition of social management. More importantly, it also offered a new set of techniques. By 1900 these techniques included birth control, segregation, sterilisation and the use of legislative measures by the state to alter the relative birth rates of the fit and unfit.

160

The second tradition associated with social hygiene was that of political economy. The precepts of political economy and health reform had always been closely entwined since the nineteenth century as recent work has shown.[1] Social hygiene adopted the idea that, in addition to physical health, it was also thrift, discipline and economic productiveness which made up fitness. The idea of health and population as economic resources also influenced social hygiene. By the twentieth century, however, capitalism had changed. Rationalisation not *laissez faire* was being considered as the key to future economic progress. This was a response to the increasing monopolisation of industry, particularly the technologically advanced industries. Social hygiene reflected these changes. A rationalised firm had to be an organised and planned enterprise, since competition alone would not ensure that the most efficient survived. Similarly, social hygienists, whilst they prized the virtues associated with *laissez-faire* capitalism, believed that the population and the birth rate must be consciously planned and managed by state policy. This was particularly so since the trend of modern legislation was to reduce the impact of economic competition through social welfare measures. In addition, monopolisation would create major structural problems. It would necessitate, so it was believed, a smaller and more productive workforce. This would exacerbate the problem of the residuum. Negative eugenics could aid the disappearance of the residuum, positive eugenics, health reform and industrial psychology could select those best fitted to take their places in the new economic order.

Therefore, the increasing concern with physical and mental fitness in the late-nineteenth and early-twentieth centuries is not simply an extension of the system of domination described by Foucault. Foucault's account gains credibility only by leaving out the political and social determinants. In fact, it reduces politics to the relationship between the individual and the ideology of power transmitted through the medical and social work regimen. There were certainly practices which arose out of social hygiene that exercised power upon the individual of a painful and distasteful kind. Or, as Foucault says, forced the individual to collaborate willingly in their own domination through the ideology of what was scientifically or socially proper for them to accept. None the less, the ideology of power cannot explain alone the historical and political determinants of the rise of social hygiene.

Limitations existed upon the influence of social hygiene for several reasons. First, governments in Britain were, except in time of acute crisis or ideological fervour, dominated by the day-to-day concerns of administration and by financial constraints. They tended, therefore, to look upon schemes of major social reconstruction with a critical eye, from whatever quarter they emanated. Governments were also reluctant to legislate in morally controversial areas. This delayed their support for birth control[2] and it prevented the acceptance of sterilisation. None the less the period 1900-39 does demonstrate an advance in the ethic of social hygiene. At the same time, by the end of the 1930s, organised resistance to social hygiene had grown — spurred on by the political and social changes of that decade. The rise of organised labour meant that whereas the elected Parliament of 1913 had been almost unanimous in their support of the Mental Deficiency Bill, it was difficult, in succeeding decades, to get that type of parliamentary support. Similarly the leftward trend among intellectuals in the 1930s, which has been alternatively exaggerated and under-appreciated by historians, clearly affected attitudes to the social issues of the time among which were explanations of the relationship between ill-health and poverty. Moreover social hygiene had always represented only one cluster of beliefs about health and welfare among many. That is why it is important to identify the institutions and social groups which attached themselves to it, for we cannot presume that social hygiene was hegemonic and therefore part of everyone's intellectual universe. In addition, there were unique historical circumstances — Imperial rivalry, the demand for national efficiency and middle-class alarm at the rise of organised labour — which brought social hygiene into existence.

However, social hygiene does appear to have struck roots in part of British society. As the 1960s drew to a close some of the same preoccupations began to surface in British social life. In 1974, the Conservative Shadow Minister of Education made a speech to his Party outlining his fears about the differential birth rate,

> The balance of our population, our human stock is threatened. A recent article in *Poverty*, published by the Child Poverty Action Group showed that a high and rising proportion of children are being born to mothers least fitted to bring children into the world and bring them up. They are born to mothers who were first pregnant in adolescence in social classes 4 and 5. Many of these girls are unmarried, many are deserted or divorced or soon will be. Some are of low intelligence, most of low educational attainment. They are unlikely to be able to give children the stable emotional background, the consistent combination of love and firmness which are more important than riches. They are producing problem children, the future unmarried mothers,

delinquents, denizens of our borstals, subnormal educational establishments, prisons, hostels for drifters . . . Single parents from classes four and five, are now producing one-third of all births. A high proportion of these births are a tragedy for the mother, the child and father.

Yet what shall we do? If we do nothing the nation moves towards degeneration . . . all the more serious, when we think of the loss of people through emigration as our semi-socialism deprives them of rewards and satisfactions. Yet proposals to extend birth control facilities . . . evoke moral opposition . . . But which is the lesser evil until we remoralise whole groups of people?[3]

The reception to this speech was generally unfavourable. It was quickly pointed out that whereas the lowest social group was producing one-third of all births, their overall birth rate was falling and falling faster than among the managerial and professional classes.[4] In the 1980s, however, the government's commitment to a balanced budget, retrenchment in welfare spending, economic individualism and deflation led to a reconsideration of social policy in the Conservative Party. The discussions taking place in 1983 suggested a number of changes in social policy. The provision of welfare, it was argued, should be shifted back onto the family, unemployment should be mitigated by encouraging married women to leave the labour market, the virtues of thrift, foresight and independence should be encouraged in the schools and birth control propaganda should be directed at those social groups most likely to be irresponsible parents with unwanted or neglected children.[5]

In a sense, therefore, this essay in the history of ideas has some contemporary relevance. Social hygiene lived, died and, possibly, rose again. The economic and social determinants of its existence and the structure of its ideas are probably of historical interest only. None the less, there are indications, at least, that social hygiene exercises a significant residual influence in thinking on British social policy.

Notes

1. See W. Coleman, *Death is a Social Disease. Public Health and Political Economy in Early Industrial France* (University of Wisconsin Press, Wisconsin, 1982) and F.B. Smith, *The People's Health, 1830-1910* (Croom Helm, London, 1982).

2. See Soloway, *Birth Control and the Population Question in England, 1877-1930* (University of North Carolina Press, Chapel Hill, 1982).

3. Sir Keith Joseph, *The Guardian*, 21 October 1974.

4. Ibid.

5. Report of a discussion in the Conservative Party's Family Policy Unit, *The Times*, 17 February 1983.

SELECT BIBLIOGRAPHY

Manuscript Sources

Political and Economic Planning Papers (PEP), London School of Economics.
National Institute of Industrial Psychology Papers (NIIP), London School of Economics.
Next Five Years Group (NFYG), Clifford Allen Papers, University of South Carolina
    at Columbia.
Eugenics Society Papers (Eug), Wellcome Institute for the History of Medicine, London,
    and the Eugenics Society Library, 69 Eccleston Square, London W1.
Penrose Papers, University College, London.
Wedgwood Papers, University of Keele, Staffs.

Government Archives, Public Record Office, Kew

Ministry of Health Files PRO MH 58/100, 101, 103, 104A
                          PRO MH 51/559
                          PRO MH 56/40
                          PRO MH 55/688
                          PRO MH 58/311
                          PRO MH 56/52
Economic Advisory Committee, Committee on Rationalisation, PRO CAB 58/175-80, Scientific Research, CP 185/34, CAB 24/250.

Official Publications

House of Commons Debates.
Royal Commission on the Care and Control of the Feebleminded, PP Cmnd 4202 and
    Cmnd 4215-4221, Vols xxiv-xxxix, 1908.
Report of the Inter-departmental Committee on Mental Deficiency, 1925-29 (Wood Report),
    3 vols, 1929.
Report of the Departmental Committee on Sterilisation (Brock Report), PP Cmnd 4485,
    vol. xv, 1934.
Report of the Royal Commission on Population, Cmnd 7695, 1949.
Royal Commission on the Law Relating to Mental Illness and Mental Deficiency, Cmnd
    169, 1956-57.
Report of the Investigation into the Industrial Conditions in Depressed Areas, Cmnd 4728,
    1934.

Other Printed Sources

Annual Report of the Central Association for Mental Welfare (CAMW).
Annual Report of the Eugenics Society.
TUC Reports.
Medical Research Council, Special Report Series.
Directory of Directors, 1908-13 and 1937.
Dictionary of Labour Biography.
Dictionary of National Biography.
Who was Who?

Periodicals

British Medical Journal.
Bulletin of the Committee against Malnutrition.
Dublin Journal of Medicine.
The Economist.
Encounter.
English Review.
Eugenics Review.
Fortnightly Review.
Journal of Heredity.
Journal of Hygiene.
Journal of Mental Hygiene.
Journal of Mental Science.
Justice.
Lancet.
Life and Letters.
Mental Welfare (previously *Studies in Mental Inefficiency, Journal of the CAMW*).
The Nation.
National Labour Newsletter.
National Review.
New Health (Journal of the New Health Society).
New Statesman.
Nineteenth Century and After.
Planning.
Political Quarterly.
Proceedings of the Royal Society of Medicine.
Progress and the Scientific Worker (bi-monthly journal of the Association of
    Scientific Workers).
Quarterly Review.
The Realist.
Saturday Review.
Spectator.
Weekend Review.

Newspapers

Daily Mail.
The Empire Citizen.
The Guardian.
Northern Whig.
The Times.
The Worker.

Printed Books and Articles

Adams, P. *Health of the State* (Praeger Special Studies in Social Welfare, New York, 1982)
Addison, P. *The Road to 1945* (Cape, London, 1975)
Allen, G. *Life Science in the Twentieth Century* (John Wiley and Sons, New York, 1975)
Allen, G.C. *The Industrial Development of Birmingham and the Black Country* (Allen and Unwin, London, 1929)

Armstrong, D. *The Political Anatomy of the Body. Medical Knowledge in Britain in the Twentieth Century* (Cambridge University Press, Cambridge, 1983)

Austoker, J.' Biological Education and Social Reform: the BSHC 1925-42', unpublished MA, University of London, 1981

Baker, J.R. and Haldane, J.B.S. *Biology in Everyday Life* (Allen and Unwin, London, 1933)

Banks, O. and Banks, J.A. *Feminism and Family Planning in Victorian England* (Liverpool University Press, Liverpool, 1964)

Barnes, G. *From Workshop to War Cabinet* (Herbert Jenkins, London, 1923)

Belfrage, H.S. *What's Best to Eat* (Heinemann, London, 1926)

Blacker, C.P. *Birth Control and the State. A Plea and a Forecast* (Kegan Paul, London, 1926)

—— *A Social Problem Group?* (Oxford University Press, Oxford, 1937)

—— *Neurosis and the Mental Health Services* (Oxford University Press, Oxford, 1946)

—— *Eugenics, Galton and After* (Duckworth, London, 1952)

Blackett, B. *A Layman's Plea for a Positive Health Policy* (British Social Hygiene Council, London, 1932)

—— *Planned Money* (Constable and Company, London, 1932)

—— 'The Era of Planning' in George R.S. Taylor (ed.), *Great Events in History* (Cassell and Company, London, 1934)

Boothby, R., MP, Macmillan, H., MP, Stanley, Hon. O., MP and Loder, J., MP *Industry and the State. A Conservative View* (Macmillan, London, 1927)

Box, J. *R.A. Fisher. The Life of A Scientist* (Wiley, New York, 1978)

Bowler, P.J. 'E.W. MacBride's Lamarckian Eugenics', *Annals of Science*, vol. 41 (1984) pp. 245-60

Bristow, E. *Vice and Vigilance, Purity Movements in Britain since 1700* (Rowman, New York, 1977)

—— *Prostitution and Prejudice. The Jewish Fight Against White Slavery, 1870-1939* (Schocken, New York, 1983)

Brockington, C.F. *A Short History of Public Health*, 2nd edn (J. and A. Churchill, London, 1966)

Burnett, J. *Plenty and Want. A Social History of Diet in England from 1815 to the Present Day* (Nelson, London, 1966)

Calder, A. *The People's War, Britain 1939-45* (Cape, London, 1969)

Carpenter, L.P. 'Corporatism in Britain 1930-45', *Journal of Contemporary History*, vol. 11 (1976) pp. 3-25

Carr Saunders, A.M. *Population* (Humphrey Milford for Oxford University Press, London, 1925)

Cathcart, E.P. *The Human Factor in Industry* (Oxford University Press, Oxford, 1928)

Cattell, R.B. *The Fight for Our National Intelligence* (P.S. King and Son Ltd, London, 1937)

—— *Human Affairs* (Macmillan, London, 1937)

Chance, W. *The Better Administration of the Poor Law* (Sonnenschein and Company, London, 1895)

—— *The Ministry of Health and the Poor Law* (P.S. King and Son Ltd, London, 1923)

—— *Old Age Pensions. The Better Way* (British Constitutional Pamphlets, no. 10, London, 1907)

Chapman, A.L. and Knight, R. *Wages and Salaries in the UK 1920-38* (Cambridge University Press, Cambridge, 1953)

Charles, E. *The Twilight of Parenthood* (Watts and Company, London, 1934)

Charles, R. *The Development of Industrial Relations, 1911-39* (Hutchinson, London, 1973)

Chesser Sloan, E. 'The Lancashire Operative', *National Review*, vol. 54 (1909), pp. 684-92

—— 'The Health of the Nation', *National Review*, vol. 56 (1911), pp. 755-62

—— *Women, Marriage and Motherhood* (Funk and Wagnall, New York, 1913)

Chick, Dame H. 'Study of Rickets in Vienna', *Medical History*, vol. 20, no. 6 (1976), pp. 41-51

Clark, C. *The National Income, 1924-31* (Macmillan, London, 1932)

Clark, R. *JBS. The Life and Work of J.B.S. Haldane* (Hodder and Stoughton, London, 1968)

Clarke, P. *Lancashire and the New Liberalism* (Cambridge University Press, Cambridge, 1971)

—— *Liberals and Social Democrats* (Cambridge University Press, Cambridge, 1978)

Coleman, W. *Death is a Social Disease. Public Health and Political Economy in Early Industrial France* (University of Wisconsin Press, Wisconsin, 1982)

Collini, S. *Liberalism and Sociology. L.T. Hobhouse and Political Argument in England 1880-1914* (Cambridge University Press, Cambridge, 1979)

D'Arcy, F. *Christian Ethics and Modern Thought* (Longmans Green and Company, London, 1912)

Davies, S.P. *Social Control of the Feebleminded* (Constable, London, 1930)

Davin, A. 'Imperialism and Motherhood', *History Workshop*, vol. 5 (1978), pp. 9-65

Dendy, M. 'On the Training and Management of Feebleminded Children' in C.P. Lapage, *Feeblemindedness in Children of School Age* (University of Manchester, Medical Series, no. 13, Manchester, 1911)

Denman, R.D. *Political Sketches* (Charles Thurman and Sons, Carlisle, 1948)

Donzelot, J. *The Policing of Families* (Pantheon, New York, 1979)

Doyal, L. with Pennell, I. *The Political Economy of Health* (Pluto, London, 1979)

Drummond, J.C. and Wilbraham, A. *The Englishman's Food: A History of Five Centuries of English Diet*, rev. edn (Jonathan Cape, London, 1957)

Dyhouse, C. 'Working Class Mothers and Infant Mortality in England, 1895-1914', *Journal of Social History*, vol. 12 (1978), pp. 248-67

Ellis, H. *The Task of Social Hygiene* (Constable, London, 1912)

—— *My Confessional* (John Lane, The Bodley Head Press, London, 1934)

Earle, F.M. *Methods of Choosing a Career* (George Harrap and Company, London, 1931)

Farrall, L.A. The Origins and Growth of the English Eugenics Movement 1865-1925, unpublished doctoral dissertation, Indiana University, 1970

—— 'The History of Eugenics. A Bibliographical Review', *Annals of Science*, vol. 36 (1979) pp. 111-23

Feldman, I. 'Population and Ideology', *History of Political Thought*, vol. 5 (1984) pp. 362-75

Finer, S.E. *The Life and Times of Sir Edwin Chadwick* (Methuen, London, 1952)

Fisher, R.A. *The Genetical Theory of Natural Selection* (Clarendon Press, Oxford, 1930)

Foucault, M. *History of Sexuality*, vol. 1 (Pantheon, New York, 1978)

Fraser, D. *The Evolution of the British Welfare State* (Macmillan, London, 1973)

Freeden, M. *The New Liberalism. An Ideology of Social Reform* (Oxford University Press, Oxford, 1978)

—— 'Eugenics and Progressive Thought. A Study in Ideological Affinity', *Historical Journal*, vol. 22 (1979) pp. 645-71

—— 'Eugenics and Ideology', *Historical Journal*, vol. 26 (1983) pp. 959-62

Gailey, A. *The Unionist Government's Policy Towards Ireland 1895-1905*, unpublished PhD thesis, University of Cambridge, Cambridge, 1982

Gilbert, B.B. 'Health and Politics. The British Physical Deterioration Report of 1904', *Bulletin of the History of Medicine*, vol. 39 (1965), pp. 143-53

—— *The Evolution of National Insurance in Great Britain* (Michael Joseph, London, 1966)

Glass, D.V. *The Struggle for Population* (Clarendon Press, Oxford, 1936)

Gray, J.L. *The Nation's Intelligence* (Watts and Company, London, 1936)
Greenwood, Major *Some Pioneers in Social Medicine* (Oxford University Press, Oxford, 1948)
Haldane, J.B.S. *The Inequality of Man* (Chatto and Windus, London, 1932)
—— *Human Biology and Politics* (British Science Guild, London, 1934)
—— *Heredity and Politics* (Allen and Unwin, London, 1938)
—— *Science and Everyday Life* (Lawrence and Wishart, London, 1939)
—— *New Paths in Genetics* (Allen and Unwin, London, 1941)
Hall, R. *Passionate Crusader. The Life of Marie Stopes* (Deutsch, London, 1977)
Halsey, A.H. 'T.H. Marshall, Past and Present, 1893-1981', *Sociology*, vol. 18 (1984), pp. 1-18
Hancock, W.K. and Gowing, M.M. *The British War Economy* (Longmans Green and Company and His Majesty's Stationery Office, London, 1949)
Harris, J. *Unemployment and Politics, 1886-1914* (Oxford University Press, Oxford, 1972)
—— *William Beveridge. A Biography* (Oxford University Press, Oxford, 1977)
Hay, J.R. *Origins of the Liberal Welfare Reforms* (Macmillan, London, 1975)
Hearnshaw, L.S. *A Short History of British Psychology, 1840-1940* (Methuen, London, 1964)
—— *Cyril Burt, Psychologist* (Hodder and Stoughton, London, 1979)
Hogben, L. *Genetic Principles in Medicine and Social Science* (Williams and Norgate, London, 1931)
—— *Nature and Nurture* (Williams and Norgate, London, 1933)
—— *The Retreat from Reason*, Conway Memorial Lecture (Walter and Company, London, 1936)
—— (ed.) *Political Arithmetic* (Allen and Unwin, London, 1938)
—— *The New Authoritarianism* (Watts and Company, London, 1949)
Honigsbaum, F. *The Division in British Medicine. The Separation of General Practice from Hospital Care 1911-68* (St. Martin's, New York, 1979)
—— *The Struggle for the Ministry of Health 1914-1919.* Occasional Papers on Social Administration, no. 37 (G. Bell and Sons, London, 1970)
Howson, S. and Winch, D. *The Economic Advisory Council, 1930-39* (Cambridge University Press, Cambridge, 1977)
Huxley, J. 'The Applied Science of the Next Hundred Years', *Life and Letters*, vol. II (1934) pp. 38-46
—— *Memories I* (Allen and Unwin, London, 1970)
Ihde, J. 'Recognition of Rickets as a Deficiency Disease, Part 1', *Pharmacy in History*, vol. 16 (1974), pp. 83-5
—— 'Recognition of Rickets as a Deficiency Disease, Part 2', *Pharmacy in History*. vol. 17 (1975), pp. 13-20
Jones, D. Caradog (ed.) *Merseyside: The Relief of the Poor* (University of Liverpool Press, Liverpool, 1936)
—— *The Social Survey of Merseyside* (Hodder and Stoughton, London, 1934)
—— *The Social Problem Group. Poverty and Subnormality of Intelligence* (Canadian Bar Association, Toronto, 1945)
Jones, G. Stedman *Outcast London* (Oxford University Press, Oxford, 1971)
Jones, G. 'British Scientists, Lysenko and the Cold War', *Economy and Society*, vol. 8 (1979), pp. 26-58
—— 'Eugenics and Social Policy Between the Wars', *Historical Journal*, vol. 25 (1982) pp. 717-28
—— *Social Darwinism and English Thought* (Harvester Press, Sussex, 1980)
Jones, K. *A History of the Mental Health Services* (Routledge and Kegan Paul, London, 1972)
Kevles, D. 'Annals of Eugenics, Parts 1-4', *The New Yorker* (8 October 1984),

pp. 51-115; (15 October 1984), pp. 52-120; (22 October 1984); pp. 92-151; (29 October 1984), pp. 51-117

Kidd, A. 'Charity Organisation and the Unemployed in Manchester, 1870-1914', *Social History*, vol. 9 (1984), pp. 45-66

Kopsch, H. 'The Approach of the Conservative Party to Social Policy during World War Two', unpublished PhD thesis, University of London, 1970

Kuczynski *Population Movements* (Clarendon Press, Oxford, 1936)

Labisch, A. 'Doctors, Workers and the Scientific Cosmology of the Industrial World', *Journal of Contemporary History*, vol. 20 (1985), pp. 599-615

Lawrence, C. 'Incommunicable Knowledge, Science, Technology and the Clinical Art in Britain 1850-1914', *Journal of Contemporary History*, vol. 20 (1985), pp. 503-20

Lewis, J. *The Politics of Motherhood* (Croom Helm, London, 1980)

—— and Brookes, B. 'The Peckham Health Centre, PEP and the Concept of General Practice during the 1930s and 1940s', *Medical History*, vol. 27 (1983) pp. 151-61

Leeper, R. 'A Note on the Causation of Insanity in Ireland', *Dublin Journal of Medicine*, vol. 123 (1912), pp. 180-7

Lidbetter, E.J. *Heredity and the Social Problem Group* (E. Arnold and Company, London, 1933)

Lowes, R.A. 'Eugenicists, Doctors and the Quest for National Efficiency, An Educational Crusade, 1900-39', *History of Education*, vol. 8 (1979), pp. 293-306

Love, R. 'Alice in Eugenics-Land', *Annals of Science*, vol. 36 (1979), pp. 145-58

Lucas, A. *Industrial Reconstruction and the Control of Competition* (Longmans Green and Company, London, 1937)

McCleary, G.F. *The Maternal and Child Welfare Movement* (P.S. King, London, 1935)

—— *The Menace of British Depopulation* (Allen and Unwin, London, 1937)

MacKenzie, D. *Statistics in Britain* (Edinburgh University Press, Edinburgh, 1981)

Mackintosh, J.M. *Trends of Opinion About the Public Health* (Oxford University Press, Oxford, 1953)

Macmillan, H. *Reconstruction. A Plea for a National Policy, London* (Macmillan, London, 1933)

—— *The Middle Way* (Macmillan, London, 1938)

—— *Winds of Change* (Macmillan, London, 1966)

McLaren, A. *Birth Control in Nineteenth-century England* (Croom Helm, London, 1978)

Macnicol, J. *The Movement for Family Allowances* (Heinemann, London, 1981)

Marshall, T.H. *Citizenship and Social Class* (Cambridge University Press, Cambridge, 1950)

Marwick, A. *Clifford Allen, the Open Conspirator* (Oliver and Boyd, Edinburgh and London, 1964)

—— 'Middle Opinion in the Thirties. Planning, Progress and Political Agreement', *English Historical Review*, vol. 79 (1964), pp. 285-98

Mayr, E. *The Growth of Biological Thought* (Belknap Press for Harvard University, Cambridge, Mass., 1982)

M'Gonigle, G.C.M. and Kirby, J. *Poverty and Public Health* (Gollancz, London, 1936)

Mommsen, W.J. (ed.), *The Emergence of the Welfare State in Britain and Germany 1850-1950* (Croom Helm, London, 1981)

Mond, A. *Industry and Politics* (Macmillan, London, 1927)

Morgan, K.O. and Morgan, J. *Portrait of a Progressive. The Political Career of Christopher, Viscount Addison* (Oxford University Press, Oxford, 1980)

—— *Labour in Power 1945-1951* (Clarendon Press, Oxford, 1984)

Mowat, C.L. *Britain Between the Wars* (University of Chicago Press, Illinois, 1955)

—— *The Charity Organisation Society 1869-1913* (Methuen, London, 1961)

Myers, C.S. *Mind and Work* (University of London Press, London, 1920)
—— *Industrial Psychology in Britain* (Jonathan Cape, London, 1927)
—— *Industrial Psychology* (Butterworth, London, 1929)
—— *Business Rationalisation* (Pitman and Sons, London, 1932)
Myers, C.S. and Welch, H.J. *Ten Years of Industrial Psychology* (Pitman and Sons, London, 1932)
Navarro, V. *Class Struggle, the State and Medicine* (Prodist, New York, 1978)
Newman, Sir G. *The Building of a Nation's Health* (Macmillan, London, 1939)
Newsholme, Sir A. *Fifty Years in Public Health* (Allen and Unwin, London, 1935)
—— *The Last Thirty Years in Public Health* (Allen and Unwin, London, 1936)
Noble, D.F. *America by Design. Science, Technology and the Rise of Corporate Capitalism* (Oxford University Press, New York, 1979)
Norton, B. 'Fisher and the Neo-Darwinian Synthesis' in E.G. Forbes (ed.), *The Human Implications of Scientific Advance* (Edinburgh University Press, Edinburgh, 1978)
Orr Boyd, J. *Food, Health and Income* (Macmillan, London, 1936)
Pater, J.E. *The Making of the National Health Service* (King's Fund Historical Series, London, 1981)
Paul, D. 'Eugenics and the Left'', *Journal of the History of Ideas*, vol. 45 (1984) pp. 561-90
Peel, J. 'Birth Control and the British Working Class Movement', *Society for the Study of Labour History*, vol. 7 (1963), pp. 16-22
Penrose, L.S. *Mental Defect* (Sidgwick and Jackson, London, 1933)
—— *Heredity and Environment in Human Affairs*. The Convocation Lecture (National Children's Home, London, 1955)
People's League of Health *The Inception of the League*, by Olga Nethersole (People's League, London, 1920)
—— *How to Feed the Family*, by Col. P.S. Lelean (People's League, London, c. 1926)
—— *The People's League of Health Lectures* (Routledge and Sons, London, 1926)
—— *Report of a Deputation of the People's League to the Minister of Health, Neville Chamberlain, 28 June 1927* (People's League, London, 4 December 1928)
Pinder, J. (ed.) *Fifty Years of Economic Planning 1931-81*, (Heinemann, London, 1981)
Pinsent, E.F. 'Social Responsibility and Heredity', *National Review*, vol. 56 (1910) pp. 506-15
Political and Economic Planning *An Enabling Act for Britain* (PEP, London, 1934)
—— *Future British Population* (PEP, London, 1934)
—— *The Malnutrition Controversy* (PEP, London, 1936)
—— *The British Health Services* (PEP, London, 1937)
—— *Population Policy* (PEP, London, 1948)
Robbins, L. *An Essay on the Nature and Significance of Economic Science* (Macmillan, London, 1932)
—— *The Great Depression* (Macmillan, London, 1934)
—— *The Economic Basis of Class Conflict and Other Essays* (Macmillan, London, 1939)
Rolfe, Neville S. *Social Biology and Welfare* (Allen and Unwin, London, 1949)
Rose, M.E. *The Relief of Poverty 1834-1914* (Macmillan, London, 1972)
Rosen, G. 'What is Social Medicine?' *Bulletin of the History of Medicine*, vol. 21 (1947), pp. 674-733
—— *A History of Public Health* (MD Monographs in Medical History, New York, 1958)
—— *Madness in Society* (Routledge, London, 1968)
Rosenberg, C.E. *No Other Gods. On Science and American Social Thought* (Johns Hopkins University Press, Baltimore, 1976)
Rubenstein, W.D. 'Wealth, Elites and the Class Structure of Modern Britain', *Past and Present*, vol. 76 (1977), pp. 99-126

—— *Men of Property, the Very Wealthy in Britain since the Industrial Revolution* (Croom Helm, London, 1981)

Ryle, J.A. *Changing Disciplines: Lectures on the History, Methods and Motives of Social Pathology* (Oxford University Press, Oxford, 1948)

Schiller, F.C.S. *Social Decay and Eugenical Reform* (Constable and Company, London, 1932)

Searle, G.R. *The Quest for National Efficiency* (Blackwell, Oxford, 1971)

—— *Eugenics and Politics in Britain, 1900-14* (Noordhof International, Leyden, 1976)

—— 'Eugenics and Politics in Britain in the 1930s', *Annals of Science*, vol. 36 (1979), pp. 159-69

—— 'The Edwardian Liberal Party and Business', *English Historical Review*, vol. 98 (1983), pp. 28-60

Semmel, B. *Imperialism and Social Reform* (Allen and Unwin, London, 1960)

Shuttleworth, G.E. *Mentally Deficient Children* (H.K. Lewis, London, 1895)

Skidelsky, R. *Politicians and the Slump* (Macmillan, London, 1967)

Smith, F.B. *The People's Health, 1830-1910* (Croom Helm, London, 1979)

Soloway, R.A. *Birth Control and the Population Question in England 1877-1930* (University of North Carolina Press, Chapel Hill, 1982)

Spence, J.C. and Charles, J.A. *Investigation into the Health and Nutrition of the Children of Newcastle-upon-Tyne between the ages of one and five years* (City and County of Newcastle-upon-Tyne, Newcastle, 1934)

Stevenson, J. *Social Conditions in Britain Between the Wars* (Penguin, Harmondsworth, 1977)

—— *British Society 1914-45* (Pelican, London, 1984)

Stevenson, J. and Cook, C. *The Slump. Society and Politics during the Depression* (Cape, London, 1978)

Sutherland, G. *Ability, Merit and Measurement* (Clarendon Press, Oxford, 1984)

Tanner, W.E. *Sir William Arbuthnot Lane* (Baillière, Tindall and Company, London, 1946)

Thane, P. *The Foundations of the Welfare State* (Longmans, London, 1982)

Thomson, J.A. 'Biology and Social Hygiene', *Quarterly Review*, vol. 246 (1926) pp. 28-48

Thomson, Sir Landsborough *Half a Century of Medical Research*, 2 vols (HMSO, London, 1970)

Thurtle, E. *Time's Winged Chariot* (Chaterson, London, 1945)

Titmuss, R.M. *Poverty and Population* (Macmillan, London, 1938)

—— *Problems of Social Policy* (Longmans Green and Company and HMSO, London, 1950)

—— *Essays on the Welfare State* (Allen and Unwin, London, 1963)

Towers, B.A. 'Health Education Policy, 1916-1926, Venereal Disease and the Prophylaxis Dilemma', *Medical History*, vol. 24 (1980), pp. 70-87

Tredgold, A.F. *Mental Deficiency* (Baillière and Company, London, 1908)

Urwick, L. *The Meaning of Rationalisation* (Nisbet and Company, London, 1929)

Vincent, A.W. 'The Poor Law Reports of 1909 and the Social Theory of the Charity Organisation', *Victorian Studies*, vol. 27 (1984), pp. 303-43

Watson, F. *Dawson of Penn* (Chatto and Windus, London, 1950)

Webster, C. (ed.) *Biology, Medicine and Society 1840-1940* (Cambridge University Press, Cambridge, 1981)

—— 'Healthy or Hungry Thirties?' *History Workshop*, vol. 13 (1982), pp. 110-29

Weiler, P. *The New Liberalism. Liberal Social Theory in Great Britain 1889-1914* (Garland, New York, 1982)

Werskey, G. *The Visible College* (Allen Lane, London, 1978)

Whetham, W.C.D. *Politics and the Land* (Cambridge University Press, Cambridge, 1927)

Wiener, M. *English Culture and the Decline of the Industrial Spirit, 1850-1980* (Cambridge University Press, Cambridge, 1981)

Willcocks, A.J. *The Creation of the National Health Service* (Routledge and Kegan Paul, London, 1967)

Winter, J.M. 'Military Fitness and Civilian Health in Britain during the First World War', *Journal of Contemporary History*, vol. 15 (1980), pp. 211-44

Woodhouse, J. 'Eugenics and the Feebleminded', *History of Education*, vol. II (1982), pp. 127-37

Wootten, B. *Plan or No Plan* (Gollancz, London, 1934)

INDEX